Impotence in Diabetes

Impotence in Diabetes

Edited by

David E Price MA, MD, FRCP
Consultant Physician and
Honorary Senior Lecturer
Morriston Hospital
Swansea
UK

William D Alexander FRCP
Consultant Physician
Diabetes Unit, Western General Hospital
Edinburgh
UK

MARTIN
DUNITZ

© 2002 Martin Dunitz Ltd, a member of the Taylor & Francis group

First published in the United Kingdom in 2002 by Martin Dunitz Ltd,
The Livery House, 7–9 Pratt Street, London NW1 0AE

Tel: +44 (0) 20 7482 2202
Fax: +44 (0) 20 7267 0159
E-mail: info@dunitz.co.uk
Website: http://www.dunitz.co.uk

A CIP record for this book is available from the British Library.

ISBN 90 5823 2077

Although every effort has been made to ensure that all owners of copyright material
have been acknowledged in this publication, we would be glad to acknowledge in
subsequent reprints or editions any omissions brought to our attention.

Distributed in the USA by
Fulfilment Center
Taylor & Francis
7625 Empire Drive
Florence, KY 41042, USA
Toll Free Tel.: +1 800 634 7064
E-mail: cserve@routledge_ny.com

Distributed in Canada by
Taylor & Francis
74 Rolark Drive
Scarborough, Ontario M1R 4G2, Canada
Toll Free Tel.: +1 877 226 2237
E-mail: tal_fran@istar.ca

Distributed in the rest of the world by
Thomson Publishing Services
Cheriton House
North Way
Andover, Hampshire SP10 5BE, UK
Tel.: +44 (0)1264 332424
E-mail: salesorder.tandf@thomsonpublishingservices.co.uk

Composition by Scribe Design, Gillingham, Kent, UK
Printed and bound in Great Britain by Biddles Ltd, Guildford and King's Lynn

Contents

Contributors   vii

Series preface   viii

Chapter 1   Impotence: The neglected complication
of diabetes   1
David E Price

Chapter 2   The pathophysiology of impotence in
diabetes mellitus   9
Marek AW Miller

Chapter 3   Epidemiology and clinical features of
erectile dysfunction in diabetes   55
William D Alexander

Chapter 4   Management of impotence in diabetes   69
*David E Price, Mitra Boollel and
Nandan Koppiker*

Chapter 5   The surgical treatment of erectile
dysfunction in the diabetic patient   109
Clive Gingell

Chapter 6 How to organise an impotence clinic   121
William D Alexander

Chapter 7 The role of the general practitioner   133
Patrick J Wright

Appendix 1   151
Appendix 2   153
Appendix 3   155
Appendix 4   159

Index   161

Contributors

William D Alexander FRCP
Consultant Physician
Diabetes Unit
Western General Hospital
Crewe Road
Edinburgh
UK

Mitra Boollel MD MRCP MBA
Pfizer Central Research
Pfizer UK
Sandwich
Kent
UK

Clive Gingell
Emeritus Consultant
Urological Surgeon
Department of Urology
Southmead Hospital
Senior Clinical Lecturer
University of Bristol
Bristol
UK

Nandan Koppiker MD MRCP
Pfizer Central Research
Pfizer UK
Sandwich
Kent
UK

Marek Miller
Department of Urology
Northampton General Hospital
Cliftonville
Northampton
UK

David E Price MA MD FRCP
Consultant Physician and
Honorary Senior Lecturer
Morriston Hospital
Swansea
UK

Patrick J Wright MB CHB MRCGP
General Practitioner in Durham
City,
Clinical Assistant in Urology at
North Durham Acute Hospital
Trust
Northern Research Fellow Centre
for Health Studies
Durham University
UK

Series preface

Advances in Diabetes is a new series of monographs, each concerned with a hot or rapidly-evolving topic in diabetes. As our understanding of the processes involved in diabetes advances, at the same time new treatments emerge. There is a space for an up-to-date series of concise texts which outline these advances and this series is aimed at specialist medical and nursing practitioners in diabetes, together with their trainees. I hope that you find this series useful and stimulating as it brings together the latest information on each topic under review.

H Jonathan Bodansky, Series Editor
The General Infirmary at Leeds, Leeds, UK

chapter 1

Impotence: The neglected complication of diabetes

David E Price

Impotence has been observed in men since ancient times. It has been surrounded by myths and taboos with much discussion in past centuries being by theologians and philosophers. It was often thought to be related to evil, magic and witchcraft. Physical treatments have been suggested for many years and have included magnetism, electricity, massage and flagellation. Over the last 30 years, however, there has been a dramatic change in attitudes. It is now recognised as a common and distressing problem that was previously neglected by the medical profession. New therapies have increased the awareness of doctors and the general public of the problem and sufferers now expect an effective treatment. Diabetologists have long ignored the problem, even though it is perhaps the commonest complication of diabetic men. Old attitudes are no longer acceptable, now there is no excuse for a diabetes service not to offer treatment for erectile dysfunction. Thus, all physicians involved in the care of diabetic patients should have an understanding of the management of impotence.

Definition and terminology

The *New Oxford Dictionary of English* defines impotent as 'power-less; lacking all strength; helpless, decrepit' and (of a male) 'unable, especially for a prolonged period, to achieve a sexual erection or orgasm'. Some would argue that the wider meaning of the word makes it particularly appropriate to imply erectile dysfunction. If a man is impotent it means he is unable to achieve an erection but is also unable to function as a man, a husband or able to procreate. Thus, the emotional force of the term conveys the seriousness of the problem. Others have suggested that if we are to treat the subject seriously we need more precise definitions and terminology. With this in mind, a consensus conference met under the auspices of the US National Institutes of Health in 1992 to discuss the issue. It agreed that the word impotence is pejorative and should be replaced with the term 'erectile dysfunction' which was defined as 'the persisting or recurring inability to achieve and/or maintain an erection sufficient for satisfactory sexual activity'.[1]

Whereas the term 'erectile dysfunction' is commonly used for research and epidemiological purposes, the old-fashioned term 'impotence' remains widely used and widely understood. For the purposes of this book, therefore, the two terms are used synonymously.

Historical and sociological attitudes to sexual function

There can be few areas of human life more governed by ignorance and prejudice than sexual function. In almost every society sexuality is controlled by social convention, taboo and law. In Western society the Christian Church has had a major influence on the development of attitudes to human sexuality. In I Corinthians 7 St Paul says of virgins: 'they careth for things of the Lord that they may be holy both in body and in spirit'. As a result of his views and other writings, virginity and celibacy were advocated as ideals by the early Christian Church. These attitudes developed over centuries and became enshrined in canon law. In 1563 Pope Pius IV issued an edict, following the Council of Trent, proclaiming it was 'better and more blessed to remain in virginity, or in celibacy, than to be united in matrimony'. The stigmatisation of all aspects of human sexuality reached a peak in the 19th century. Even the medical profession shared these widely held beliefs. Sex for any purpose other than reproduction was condemned as 'conjugal onanism' by many doctors.[2]

Historical attitudes to impotence

In view of widespread attitudes to sexuality in the 18th and 19th centuries, it is perhaps not surprising that impotence was generally considered a 'divine curse'.[3] By the middle of the 19th century attitudes had changed but had scarcely become more enlightened. For the second half of that century medical writings seem obsessed that masturbation was the cause of most of men's ills and impotence in particular. In 1864 a certain Willard Parker MD coined the term 'pathological spermatorrhoea' to describe masturbation and nocturnal emissions.[4] Parker described how boys or men suffering from this condition became 'enfeebled both intellectually and physically... And became the subjects of our lunatic asylums'. He was by no means alone in his thinking; his views were representative of those of many of the medical profession at the time. In 1883 William Hammond, a former Surgeon General of the United States Army and Professor of Diseases of the Mind and Nervous System at the New York Graduate Medical School, attributed the high incidence of impotence among Victorian men to 'spermatorrhoea'. He reported fewer than 5% of men at 60 experienced satisfactory intercourse.[5] Left untreated, Hammond believed, spermatorrhoea resulted in 'total and sometimes permanent impotence'.

To prevent the curse of masturbation many solutions were suggested. Dr Frank Glenn MD of Nashville believed that boys should be circumcised at birth as it 'deprives the boy of that redundant prepuce with which he titillates the glans penis in masturbation'.[6]

Views based on such ignorance couldn't last for ever and eventually more enlightened attitudes surfaced in the medical literature. In 1899 the psychologist and radical thinker William Havelock Ellis wrote, of the received wisdom concerning masturbation, 'It seems to me that this field has rarely been viewed in a scientifically sound and morally sane light'.[7] These words could be applied to much of what has been written on impotence and male sexuality up to the 1970s.

Early research into impotence

To those thinkers who were able to see beyond impotence as a 'divine curse' or the result of 'bodily self abuse' the mind played an important role in the cause of impotence. It was Freud who popularised the importance of the psyche and learned events on the development of sexuality. In 1926 Wilhelm Stekel published a classic work elaborating the importance of psychological causes of impotence.[8] Indeed the role of psychological factors has been known for much longer. In 1500 BC Melampus of Amyththaon, a renowned physician cured Iphiclus, son of the king of Thessalia, of his impotence using an early form of psychotherapy.[9]

Throughout most of the 20th century it was the received wisdom that impotence was largely due to psychological factors: this attitude dominated even though there was little controlled evidence to support it. Erectile dysfunction was not systematically studied until Masters and Johnson undertook their seminal work in the 1950s. In their original series of over 200 impotent men they reported fewer than 5% had a physical cause for their problem.[10] This work was extended to all areas of erectile dysfunction and for the next two decades medical schools all over the world taught that 'impotence was psychogenic in origin in 95% of cases'.

The neglected complication of diabetes

Even though Masters and Johnson studied a population very different to that seen in any diabetic clinic, it was soon widely accepted that even in diabetic men impotence usually had a psychogenic cause. As no research had been done in impotent diabetic men, the findings of Masters and Johnson were simply extrapolated to diabetes. Thus, in the *Oxford Textbook of Medicine* as recently as 1987, it was stated that 'in diabetes impotence of higher central nervous origin is much commoner than organic impotence'.[11] As a result of such attitudes, treating impotence became entirely the domain of psychologists and psychosexual counsellors and was largely ignored by diabetologists.

Even as late as 1990 impotence remained the most neglected complication of diabetes even though it was widely recognised to affect over 35% of diabetic men.[12] In the United Kingdom, the British Diabetic Association (BDA) seems to have completely ignored erectile dysfunction until the 1990s. The BDA's guidelines outlining the care a diabetic patient should expect, published in 1990, makes no mention of the problem.[13] The audit guidelines produced by the same organisation in 1992 detailed every conceivable aspect of diabetes except impotence.[14]

Attitudes to erectile dysfunction in diabetes changed when effective physical treatments became available. Intracavernosal injection therapy was first described in 1982[15] and vacuum devices in 1987.[16] Overnight, simple effective treatments became available which any physician could use. These treatments worked on impotent diabetic men who had not responded to psychosexual counselling. Gradually the light dawned, as the medical profession realised at last that erectile dysfunction usually had a physical cause and required a physical treatment.

After effective treatments became available, attitudes rapidly changed, and there was a rapid upsurge of interest in the management of impotence in diabetes. However, few academic departments showed any interest in research into impotence in diabetes and, initially, there was little involvement from the pharmaceutical industry.

It was therefore left to interested clinicians to develop the management of erectile dysfunction. As a result, few controlled trials were done and the newly available physical treatments for impotence were not put to the sort of rigorous evaluation any new drug would have been. Nevertheless, diabetologists took advantage of the new treatments for impotence, and within a short space of time most diabetic units were offering treatments for erectile dysfunction. A survey of diabetologists in the UK in 1996 revealed that 96% believed that a diabetes service should manage erectile dysfunction and that almost 50% of units were treating impotence themselves (O'Malley and Price 1996, unpublished data). This represented a significant change in attitudes in a short space of time.

References

1. NIH Consensus Conference. Impotence. NIH Consensus Development Panel on Impotence. JAMA 1993; 270(1):83–90.
2. Hall LA. Forbidden by God, despised by men: masturbation, medical warnings, moral panic, and manhood in Great Britain, 1850–1950. J Hist Sexual 1992; 2:365–87.
3. Mumford KJ. 'Lost manhood': male sexual impotence and Victorian culture in the United States. J Hist Sexual 1998; 3:33–57.
4. Parker W. Spermatorrhoea. Am Med Times 1864; 8:265.
5. Hammond WA. Some remarks on sexual excesses in adult life as a cause of impotence. Va Med Monthly 1883; 10(145):150.
6. Glenn WF. Impotence in the male. Trans Tenn State Med Assoc 1892;77–93.
7. Havelock Ellis W. Auto-eroticism. Philadelphia: FA Davis & Co, 1910.
8. Steckel W. Impotence in the Male. New York: Boni and Liveright, 1927.
9. Papageorgiou MG. Forms of psychotherapy in use in ancient Greece and among the population of modern Greece. Psychother Psychsom 1969; 17:114–18.
10. Masters WH, Johnson VE. Human Sexual Inadequacy. London: Churchill, 1970.
11. Alberti KGMM, Hockaday TDR. Diabetes mellitus. In: Weatherall DJ, Ledingham JGG, Warrell DA, ed. Oxford Textbook of Medicine. Oxford: Oxford Medical Publications, 1987: 9.51–108.
12. Price D, O'Malley BP, James MA et al. Why are impotent diabetic men not being treated. Pract Diabet 1991; 8:10–11.

13. British Diabetic Association. What diabetic care to expect. Diabet Med 1990; 7:554.
14. Williams DR. A proposal for continuing audit of diabetes services. Home and Members of a Working Group of the Research Unit of the Royal College of Physicians and British Diabetic Association. Diabet Med 1992; 9(8):759–64.
15. Virag R. Intracavernous injection of papaverine for erectile failure. Lancet 1982; 2(8304):938.
16. Cooper AJ. Preliminary experience with a vacuum constriction device (VCD) as a treatment for impotence. J Psychosom Res 1987; 31(3):413–18.

chapter 2

The pathophysiology of impotence in diabetes mellitus

Marek AW Miller

Introduction

The aim of this chapter is to provide the reader with a clear under-standing of the physiology of normal penile erection and the patho-physiology of erectile dysfunction in diabetes mellitus. Many recent advances have furthered our understanding of the physiology of this facet of male sexual function and the abnormalities that contribute to the development of male erectile dysfunction in diabetes mellitus are reviewed. Many of the processes that are the basis of erectile dys-function in non-diabetic men are responsible but are accentuated in the diabetic; therefore, these pathophysiological elements will be reviewed as they are relevant to diabetes. It will be seen that neuro-pathy and angiopathy are the two most important elements in the pathophysiology of male erectile dysfunction in diabetes.

Physiology of normal penile erection

Penile erection is predominantly a vascular event. Investigations in human and animal models have shown that both erection and detumescence are haemodynamic events regulated by the state of relaxation or contraction of penile smooth muscle. This, in turn, is controlled by the autonomic nervous system. There is now widespread consensus that trabecular smooth muscle and arteriolar relaxation are the key events that initiate and control erection.[1,2] The precise mechanisms by which this occurs remain to be fully elucidated and much research effort is currently being invested into understanding the control of penile smooth muscle tone. An understanding of the anatomy of the penis is necessary before any discussion of the pathophysiology of penile erection.

Penile anatomy

The erectile tissues of the penis are found in the paired corpora cavernosa and the single corpus spongiosum. The corpus spongiosum is a ventrally situated structure that surrounds the urethra and dilates distally to form the glans penis. The paired corpora cavernosa are dorsally situated structures that are joined by a thin fibrous midline septum. The corpora cavernosa separate proximally to form the crura of the penis, which are attached to the inferior aspect of each ipsilateral ischiopubic ramus. The crura are covered inferiorly by the ischiocavernosus muscle. The bulb of the penis is situated medially between the crura and is traversed by the urethra. The bulb is firmly connected to the perineal membrane and is covered on its inferior aspect by the bulbocavernosus muscle. Each cavernosal body terminates within the glans penis, which thus forms a cap overlying them.

Each corpus is ensheathed by a thick, two-layered fibrous sheath, the tunica albuginea (Fig. 2.1) which is composed of bundles of collagen and elastin fibres. The deep fibres of the tunica albuginea pass circularly around each corpus cavernosum to unite in the midline, thus forming the pectiniform septum of the penis. The septum is incomplete distally in that it is fenestrated, such an arrangement is important for the free communication of blood flow between the

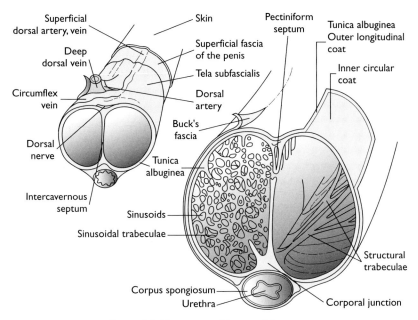

Figure 2.1 *The structural layers of the penis.*

paired erectile chambers. The outermost fibres of the tunica albuginea are longitudinally arranged and form a covering around both corpora cavernosa. In addition, all three corporeal bodies are covered by deep and superficial fascial layers that are continuous with the fascia of the perineum.

The corporeal parenchyma consists of a trabecular meshwork formed by smooth muscle fibre bundles, endothelial cells, fibroblasts and a collagenous extracellular matrix. It is this criss-crossing pattern that creates the vascular spaces known as lacunar spaces or sinusoids, which are lined by endothelial cells and surrounded in turn by smooth muscle cells. It is this arrangement which accounts for the spongy nature of the penile tissues. Immunohistochemical studies have provided some insight into the nature of the corporeal extracellular matrix. There is an abundance of types I and IV collagen with a decreased amount of type III.[3] The abundance of type IV collagen is related to the prevalence of endothelial cells within the trabeculae of

11

the corpus cavernosum. Endothelial cells are known to secrete type IV collagen, which forms the basement membrane of blood vessels.[4] These histological observations suggest that human erectile tissue may be considered as being a specialised vascular tissue.[5-7]

Electron microscopy studies investigating the ultrastructure of the erectile tissues have demonstrated the presence of gap junctions in the human corpus cavernosum.[8] It has subsequently been postulated that these gap junctions are responsible for the rapid transmission of neural or hormonal stimulation, which enables the human corpus cavernosum to behave as a coordinated functional syncytium.[9] Furthermore, electrophysiological investigations have demonstrated that human corporeal smooth muscle cells in culture are coupled by gap junctions, as shown in Fig. 2.2.[10]

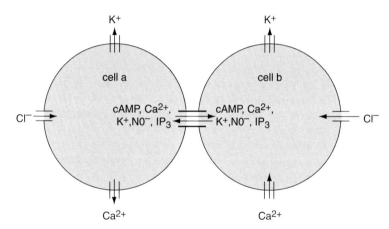

Figure 2.2 *Transmembrane channels believed to be present in the corporeal smooth muscle. Reproduced with permission.*[179]

Penile arterial supply

The blood supply to the erectile tissues is derived from the penile artery, a branch of the internal pudendal artery, which in turn is a branch of the internal iliac artery. In the anterior perineum the penile artery gives rise to a number of branches on each side: the spongiosal, bulbar or bulbourethral, the dorsal, and the deep or cavernous arteries.[11] Each cavernous artery penetrates the tunica albuginea and gives off multiple terminal helicine arteries which open directly into the sinusoidal spaces. The cavernous or deep artery frequently varies in number, origin and communication with other penile arteries.[12,13] The dorsal artery runs between the tunica albuginea and Buck's fascia with the deep dorsal vein. More distally the dorsal artery anastomoses with the spongiosal artery to form a rich arch which gives supply to the glans. It gives circumflex branches to the mid-dorsal corpora cavernosa.[14,15]

Penile venous drainage

The penis has a rich venous drainage (Fig. 2.3), which has been described in terms of deep, intermediate and superficial systems.[1] The peripheral sinusoidal spaces of the corpora cavernosa are drained by small venules that coalesce to form venous plexuses beneath the tunica albuginea. A number of these subtunical plexuses unite and

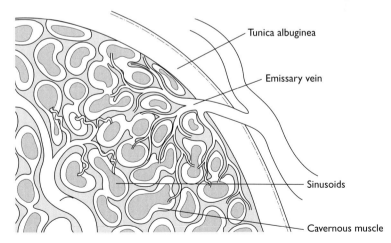

Figure 2.3 *Diagram of penile venous drainage in the flaccid state. The arteries, arterioles and sinusoids are contracted. The venous plexuses are open with free flow to the emissary veins. Reproduced with permission.*[16]

drain into the short emissary veins, which pass through the tunica albuginea.[16] In the distal, pendulous part of the penis the blood draining via the emissary veins drains laterally into circumflex veins, dorsally into dorsal veins and ventrally into urethral veins. Most of these then run into the deep dorsal vein to drain to the vesicoprostatic plexus of Santorini and the internal pudendal veins.

The deep dorsal vein drains the glans penis. The corpus spongiosum drains into both the deep dorsal vein and the internal pudendal vein. In the proximal part, or root of the penis, emissary veins drain into the cavernous and crural veins, and these drain in turn into the internal pudendal veins.

Penile nerve supply

The sacral autonomic innervation and higher centres which modulate the basic sexual reflexes are both essential for normal penile erection. The central mechanisms responsible for penile erection are not discussed here and the reader is referred elsewhere.[17] Penile erection depends on the integrated action of the sympathetic and parasympathetic systems (Fig. 2.4).

Afferent pathways
Sensory information from the penis is carried in afferents in the dorsal nerve of the penis, which then continues as the pudendal nerve to enter the sacral cord via the dorsal roots of the second and fourth segments. Sensory information is then transmitted to the cerebral cortex and thalamus in ascending tracts. Afferent input via this pathway is important in eliciting reflexogenic erections.[18,19] Recent studies have shown that in rats the cavernous nerves also contain somatic afferent fibres.[20]

Efferent pathways
Somatic efferents to the bulbocavernosus and ischiocavernosus muscles originate within the cerebral cortex, and are conveyed in the

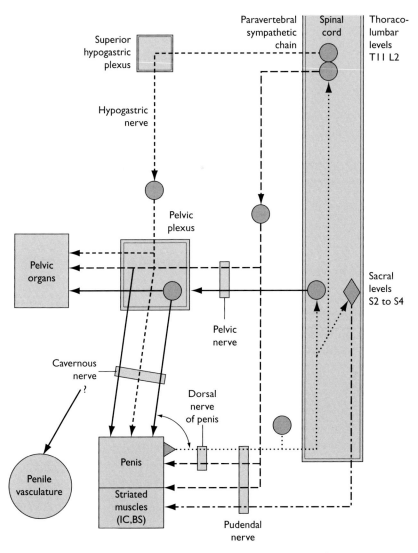

Figure 2.4 *The peripheral neural pathways involved in the control of penile erection. IC, ischiocavernosus; BS, bulbocavernosus. Reproduced with permission.*[180]

corticospinal tracts to the ventral horn of the sacral spinal cord. They synapse in the ventral horn, and large myelinated fibres travel via the anterior sacral roots (S2–S4) to join the pudendal nerve, which supplies the pelvic floor muscles. The autonomic pathways supplying the penis originate in the hippocampus, anterior cingulate gyrus and the thalamus. The fibres then pass down to the spinal erectile centres. A sacral parasympathetic erection centre lies at S2–S4 and a thoraco-lumbar sympathetic erection centre at T12–L3. From both these centres, fibres pass to the hypogastric and pelvic plexi, before fusing to form the cavernous nerves. Parasympathetic preganglionic input to the human penis originates from spinal segments S2–S4, with the cell bodies located within the intermediolateral cell column. The dendritic projections of these neurones are such that they can receive sensory input from both visceral and somatic structures.

The cavernous nerves travel along the posterolateral surface of the prostate and curve anteriorly to join the membranous urethra, and pierce the urogenital diaphragm to pass through the tunica albuginea to supply the corpora.[21] The cavernous nerves are the final common pathway for both vasodilator and vasoconstrictor neural input to the cavernous spaces in man.[22]

Haemodynamics of erection

During flaccidity (and detumescence) adrenergic sympathetic tone dominates and the terminal arterioles and sinusoidal smooth muscles are contracted.[23] Nevertheless, a small amount of arterial blood flows via the sinusoidal spaces to provide the penile nutritional requirements. The key event in penile erection is a parasympathetically-mediated (S2–4) relaxation of the blood vessels and sinusoids of the smooth muscle of the corpora cavernosa, which produces dilatation and engorgement of the sinusoids because of increased arterial inflow.[24,25] The muscle relaxation increases sinusoidal compliance and is thus able to cause elongation, expansion and erection of the penis. At erection the flow in the cavernous artery decreases and intra-cavernosal pressure rises to some 10–20 mmHg below systolic. In contrast, blood flow continues to be higher in the glans penis and corpus spongiosum.[1] There is normally some arterial inflow during systole and an absence of diastolic flow. However, during full rigidity the intracavernous pressure rises above systolic and, consequently, there is no inflow of blood.

Vascular studies have shown that a restriction of penile venous outflow is an essential component for the initiation and maintenance of a rigid erection.[26] Veno-occlusion is a passive, mechanical event that is dependent on an adequate arterial inflow, an intact tunica albuginea and a sufficient degree of smooth muscle relaxation.[16] During flaccidity the contracted trabecular smooth muscle allows for unhindered venous drainage via the subtunical venous plexus and emissary veins. During tumescence there is smooth muscle relaxation and the lacunar spaces fill with blood.[16,27] This results in the compression of the subtunical venous plexus, hence increasing the resistance to blood flow through these vessels and stopping flow in the emissary veins (Fig. 2.5). Erection is maintained by this greatly decreased venous outflow and rigidity is imparted by the rise in intracavernosal pressure, further aided perhaps by the contraction of the bulbocavernosus and ischiocavernosus muscles.[27] Thus, the veno-occlusive mechanism depends largely on adequate penile smooth muscle relaxation mediated by both

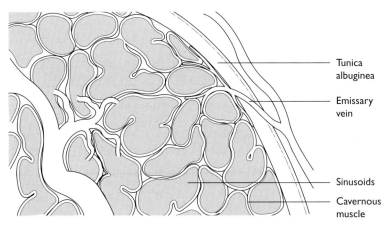

Tunica albuginea

Emissary vein

Sinusoids

Cavernous muscle

Figure 2.5 *The penis in the erect state showing the relaxed trabeculae and arterioles that allow for the blood flow into the sinusoidal spaces. The larger venules are compressed between the sinusoidal wall and the tunica albuginea. Reproduced with permission.*[16]

neurogenic and endothelial-derived elements. With the advent of rigidity, the extra-tunical deep venous system is compressed by Buck's fascia. Defects in any of the components of this mechanism can lead to the inability of the penis to 'trap' blood effectively.

Neurophysiology and pharmacology of erection

Penile erection can no longer be regarded as the result of a simple balance between pro-erectile parasympathetic activity and anti-erectile sympathetic innervation: erection is the result of parasympathetic release of acetylcholine, whereas noradrenaline release from sympathetic nerve fibres maintains flaccidity. In addition to noradrenaline and acetylcholine, a large number of putative neurotransmitters have been demonstrated in perivascular nerves, and the principal neurotransmitter has been established as nitric oxide.

The search for a single relaxant neurotransmitter in erection has been long and it seems that erection is a complicated event with much interplay and modulation between a number of neurotransmitters. Following advances in vascular physiology[28–30] it is perhaps not surprising that nitric oxide (NO) has been implicated as being the final determinant in the erectile process.[31] Nevertheless, a considerable effort continues into the elucidation of the contribution of other substances.

Adrenergic mechanisms

The sympathetic division of the autonomic nervous system has an anti-erectile effect. For example, in rabbits the stimulation of the sympathetic trunk causes the penis to shrink.[32] In man, evidence for an anti-erectile pathway comes from experiments on the actions of drugs given intracavernosally.[33] This evidence makes it almost certain that there is an anti-erectile pathway, which is continuously active when the penis is flaccid.[33] The peripheral endings of this pathway release noradrenaline, but little is known about the anatomy of the pathway.

Recently it has been proposed that there exists a pro-erectile sympathetic pathway. In the rabbit, cat and man the hypogastric plexus contains efferent nerve fibres that cause erection and tumescence. It has been shown conclusively that these fibres exist in the rabbit, and that their electrical stimulation causes erection.[32] In man, one small study reported that stimulation of the intact hypogastric plexus caused full erection in two out of nine patients and tumescence in the other seven.[34] Loss of the parasympathetic erectile pathway with survival of the sympathetic is seen in men with complete lesions of the cauda equina or conus medullaris – a proportion of these men are capable of penile erection.

Adrenergic nerves have been demonstrated in trabecular smooth muscle and in the cavernosal and helicine arteries.[35–37] It is generally accepted that in flaccidity the penile smooth muscle is contracted by noradrenaline release acting via postjunctional alpha adrenoceptors on the cavernous and helicine arteries as well as on trabecular smooth muscle.[38] Furthermore, noradrenaline release is modulated by presynaptic alpha$_2$ adrenoceptors.[38] Modulation of adrenergic activity seems to be one of the most important means by which the contractile state of the smooth muscle of the corpus cavernosum and the penile vasculature is influenced.

Noradrenaline and phenylephrine will produce concentration-dependent contraction in isolated human corpus cavernosum, corpus spongiosum, penile arteries and veins, in vivo.[36,39,40] Both the alpha$_1$ and alpha$_2$ agonists will contract trabecular tissue; however, the alpha$_2$ agonist (clonidine) was less potent in this respect.[41–43] In cavernosal artery segments, clonidine was a much more powerful contractile agent.[41] It was also shown that the alpha$_1$ blocker prazosin but not the alpha$_2$ blockers yohimbine or rauwolscine relaxed noradrenaline-precontracted trabecular tissue.[41,43] Prazosin and rauwolscine relaxed noradrenaline-induced contractions equally in cavernosal artery segments. Prazosin was more potent than rauwolscine in inhibiting contractions evoked by electrical nerve stimulation of trabecular tissue.[41,44] In arterial segments, rauwolscine was more potent than prazosin.[44] These findings suggest that alpha$_1$ adrenoceptors predominate in the human corpus cavernosum, whereas alpha$_2$ receptors predominate in the cavernosal artery. It is also known that both alpha$_1$- and alpha$_2$-adrenoceptor functions can be demonstrated in circumflex veins and the deep dorsal penile vein.[45,46] More recently, three subtypes of alpha$_1$-adrenergic receptors in mRNA (alpha$_{1A}$, alpha$_{1B}$, and alpha$_{1C}$) have been identified in human corporeal tissue. The alpha$_{1A}$ and alpha$_{1C}$ receptors were found to be the predominant subtypes expressed in this tissue at an mRNA level.[47]

The in vivo results have been confirmed by the intracavernosal injection of alpha-adrenoceptor antagonists – thus, injection of phenoxybenzamine, phentolamine and thymoxamine produced erection and tumescence[33,48] and injection of the alpha-adrenoceptor agonists metaraminol and noradrenaline caused detumescence.[49,50] It was further shown that the injection of the selective alpha$_2$-adrenoceptor blocker idazoxan had no effect, therefore supporting the view that it is the alpha$_1$ adrenoceptor that is the functionally dominant subtype.

Drugs such as trazodone and ketanserin have been reported to influence, at least partly, penile erectile tissues by the blockade of alpha adrenoceptors. Trazodone is a non-tricyclic antidepressant which was shown to have marked alpha-adrenoceptor blocking activity[50,51] and was reported to cause priapism during treatment for depressive disorders.[52] Ketanserin, a selective 5-hydroxytryptamin (5HT)-receptor blocker, which also blocks alpha adrenoceptors in human corpus cavernosum tissue, produced erection following its intracavernosal injection in man[53]. Thus, from the above, it is clear that alpha antagonism causes tumescence and erection, while alpha agonism maintains flaccidity. It has been postulated that in some cases impotence may be secondary to changes in alpha-adrenoceptor function. A small, but significant, difference was found between cavernous tissue from diabetic and non-diabetic patients with impotence. Diabetic patients had both increased and reduced sensitivity to phenylephrine.[43] In contrast, no differences were found in sensitivity to phenylephrine between cavernous tissue preparations taken from impotent men with diabetes, alcoholism, or Peyronie's disease and men with no obvious condition causing impotence.[54]

Cholinergic mechanisms

The parasympathetic autonomic nervous system has been believed to be the sole effector of physiological erections for many years. Early animal experiments showed that electrical stimulation of the nervi erigentes brought about penile erection; it was noted that this response was not abolished by atropine.[55–57] It was later suggested that a balance exists between adrenergic anti-erectile and cholinergic pro-erectile activity.[58] The function of cholinergic activity is to inhibit (via muscarinic receptors) the adrenergically induced penile flaccidity.[41,59,60] However, the exact roles of cholinergic mechanisms are unclear; indeed, a considerable body of evidence exists to suggest that vasodilatation, and hence tumescence and penile erection, are not accounted for by a simple mechanism of acetylcholine release acting via muscarinic receptors.

Muscarinic receptors have been identified in human corpus cavernosum in ligand-binding studies and have been suggested to be of M_2 and M_3 type in both cavernosal tissue and endothelium.[35,60] Furthermore, acetylcholinesterase-containing nerves have been demonstrated in human and rat penile tissue as has choline uptake, acetylcholine synthesis and release following electrical stimulation of nerves in cavernous smooth muscle.[60–62] However, there have been conflicting findings in experiments on corpus cavernosum in vitro. Some investigators report contraction of penile tissue by acetylcholine.[63] Others have found relaxation of corpus cavernosum and corpus spongiosum produced by acetylcholine when the tissue had been precontracted with noradrenaline, a response blocked by scopolamine and thus presumably mediated via muscarinic receptors.[38,59,64] Muscarinic-receptor blockade in dogs with atropine caused no effect or significant decrease in blood-flow response to pelvic nerve stimulation; however, it did curtail the erectile response.[65]

Similarly, a reduced erectile response was found in response to neurostimulation after the injection of acetylcholine, but it is unclear if this was mediated by muscarinic or alpha-adrenoceptor blockade.[66] The intracavernous injection of acetylcholine in monkeys will produce a triphasic response, including full erection.[67] The observed differences may be explained on the basis of species variation in part, but there remains a general agreement that atropine will only partially block erectile responses. Furthermore, it is also known that atropine injection fails to block penile erection in humans; this led to the suggestion that muscarinic transmission plays no significant part in penile erection.[33,68] It is noteworthy that acetylcholine release and synthesis were found to be significantly reduced in corporeal tissue from men with diabetes.[59] The destruction of the endothelium with detergent effectively eliminated/attenuated the relaxation produced by acetylcholine,[69] a finding which suggests that, as in other vascular preparations, the effect of acetylcholine is endothelium-dependent.[29]

It should be remembered that parasympathetic activity does not equate to the sole actions of acetylcholine; clearly other transmitters may be released from cholinergic nerves. There are three distinct mechanisms by which parasympathetic activity may affect erection and tumescence:

1. the release of noradrenaline may be inhibited by stimulation of muscarinic receptors on adrenergic nerve terminals;
2. the postjunctional effects of noradrenaline may be counteracted by muscarinic receptor-mediated release of relaxant factor(s) from the endothelium; and
3. the postjunctional effects of noradrenaline may be counteracted by other relaxant factors, notably NO and vasoactive intestinal polypeptide (VIP), released from the parasympathetic nerves.

Overall, parasympathetic activity contributes to penile tumescence and erection by mechanisms that antagonise the anti-erectile effects of noradrenaline. This is likely to include the muscarinic receptor-mediated inhibition of adrenergic activity as well as the generation of NO by the endothelium. Recent research efforts have focused on the role of other putative neurotransmitter substances and the term non-adrenergic non-cholinergic (NANC) transmission is used to describe these processes that are responsible for the control of penile smooth muscle relaxation.

Nitric oxide and the role of the endothelium

The vasodilatory effects of nitrates have been studied for decades; however, that endothelial cells can release a substance which causes vasodilatation was only recently discovered. It was found that the relaxation of aortic sections in response to agonists would only occur in the presence of an intact endothelium.[28] It was proposed that endothelial cells produce an endothelium-derived relaxing factor (EDRF) responsible for relaxation of vascular smooth muscle.[28] EDRF was later characterised as nitric oxide (NO); it was demonstrated that NO is formed by the action of nitric oxide synthase (NOS), an enzyme present in the vascular endothelium.[30] It was realised that NO was a secretory product of considerable import and it has become apparent that NO is a remarkable molecule with a range of biological activities including neurotransmission, vasodilatation and cytotoxicity.[70]

The sinusoidal spaces and penile vessels are lined with endothelial cells;[36,71] given the above, the role of the endothelium in erection has perhaps been neglected. It was shown that acetylcholine-induced relaxation depends on endothelial integrity and it was argued that the endothelium plays a role in the regulation of local penile haemodynamics.[71] Furthermore, it was thought that cavernosal endothelial cells may be directly innervated. This led to speculation that after the initiation of vasodilatation and increased blood flow, an additional mechanism – mediated by the endothelium – is required to maintain tumescence. The increased flow and shear forces may provide the stimulus for such a mechanism to come into operation. In addition, substance P, 5HT, acetylcholine and adenosine triphosphate (ATP) are all released from vascular beds and/or endothelial cells in culture under hypoxia-induced vasodilatation or shear stress.[72] Clearly the role of the endothelium and its stores of vasoactive agents in erectile vasodilatation cannot be ignored and warrants careful consideration.

In addition to its effects on cavernosal smooth muscle cells to produce relaxation and vasodilatation, NO also acts as both a central and peripheral neurotransmitter. Thus, penile erection is an interesting example of NO functioning as both a neurotransmitter and a vasodilator. It is thought that most penile NO is of neuronal origin[73]

23

and a number of lines of evidence show that neuronal NO is important in mediating penile erection:

1. Isolated corporeal smooth muscle strips relax when electrically stimulated, a response blocked by NO inhibitors.[69,74,75] L-arginine analogues inhibit NOS and inhibit the relaxation of cavernous tissues by electrical field stimulation and muscarinic receptor stimulation.[74,76–79]

2. Immunohistochemical studies have demonstrated NOS in the nerves of the pelvic plexus, the cavernous nerve and the processes extending into the corpora cavernosa to innervate the penile arteries in rats.[31] Furthermore, the same workers demonstrated NOS in human urogenital tissue: NOS was present in the cavernous nerves and the terminals ending in the corpus cavernosum as well as in the branches of the dorsal penile nerve.[80]

3. Electrical stimulation of the pelvic nerves of rats in vivo causes a 'physiological' erection which can be completely blocked by NOS inhibitors.[31]

Nitric oxide diffuses into cells and activates soluble guanylate cyclase, the enzyme responsible for the conversion of guanosine triphosphate to cyclic guanosine monophosphate (cGMP), thus raising the tissue levels of cGMP.[7,74,81,82] This was first demonstrated in rabbit corpus cavernosum, where it was further shown that a selective inhibition of the cGMP-specific phosphodiesterase (PDE) enhanced the relaxant effect of electrical stimulation.[74,77,81,83] Thus, the intracellular levels of this second messenger molecule are regulated by its generation via guanylate cyclase and its subsequent degradation by PDE.

It is interesting to note that NOS activity, and hence NO production, depends on O_2 tension; hence in the flaccid state, where contraction of the helicine vessels and corporeal tissues is maintained, a lowered O_2 tension might lead to lowered NOS activity, and vice versa during erection.[84,85]

In summary, there is good evidence that NO is one of the most important neurotransmitters responsible for penile erection; in this respect it is interesting that mice which lack neuronal NOS are not only viable but that they are also fertile.[86] Clearly this means that there are other pathways in existence which can mediate erection, although more recently it is thought that there may be other forms of NOS.

The potential role of other mediators

Vasoactive intestinal polypeptide

VIP is a potent vasodilator which inhibits contractile activity in many types of smooth muscle.[87] It interacts with a specific receptor and its mode of action is dependent upon the production of cyclic adenosine monophosphate (cAMP) and/or cGMP[88,89] as well as the modulation of NO release;[90] data relating to the penis suggest that VIP acts via cAMP.[91] VIP has been found in high concentrations in the erectile tissues of the human penis, in autonomic nerve fibres, penile arteries, arterioles and also circumflex veins.[37,92,93] It has long been proposed as one of the important mediators of erection, but support for this has perhaps declined in recent years following the discovery of NO.[94] Nevertheless, a number of investigators have reported that the intracavernosal injection of VIP, and more recently VIP in combination with phentolamine, does result in penile erection.[95,96] This therapeutic use of VIP lends further indirect support for the importance of its contribution as a potential neurotransmitter in normal physiological erection.

Prostaglandins

A number of studies established that the human penis can produce and metabolise prostaglandins (PGs).[97–99] Homogenates of human corpora cavernosa can produce PGE_2, $PGF_{2\text{-alpha}}$, PGD_2, and 6-keto-$PGF_{1\text{-alpha}}$ in vitro.[97] Furthermore, in the human penis it was shown that the production of PGI_2 was under, at least in part, muscarinic control.[99] Other workers demonstrated that human corpus cavernosal endothelial cells in culture also have the ability to produce 6-keto-$PGF_{1\text{-alpha}}$, PGE_2 and $PGF_{2\text{-alpha}}$.[71] The prostanoids so produced are broken down by PG 15-hydroxydehydrogenase.[98]

A role for PGs in erection was first indicated by Klinge and Sjostrand when they reported that $PGF_{2-alpha}$ contracted the corpus cavernosum and penile artery of bulls.[100] Experiments with tissue strips elucidated the ability of the various prostanoids to either contract or relax penile tissue in organ bath preparations. $PGF_{2-alpha}$, PGI_2, PGE_2 and thromboxane A_2 (TXA_2) analogues were all able to contract corpus cavernosum and arteries.[101] Jeremy et al. showed that muscarinic receptor stimulation caused prostacyclin (PGI_2) production by the human corpora cavernosa.[99] However, a major role for PGI_2 in the erectile response seems unlikely, because although PGI_2 is able to relax segments of penile vessels it was unable to relax trabecular tissue.[101] It may be argued that PGI_2 is important in the initial phases of erection to facilitate an increased blood flow as well as acting to prevent platelet aggregation in a situation of relative stasis,[101] but one must remember that this is also probably a function of NO.[102]

In organ bath experiments PGE_1 and PGE_2 were effective in relaxing human trabecular tissue as well as segments of cavernous artery.[101] PGE_1 was found to inhibit noradrenaline release from penile adrenergic nerves[103] and it had been previously shown that this PG will affect cAMP formation;[104] however, the precise intracellular mode of action and signal transduction mechanism for PGE_1 remains unclear. There is recent evidence that PGE_1 also affects intracellular calcium ion fluxes.[105] In isolated human corpus cavernosal cells, patch-clamp analysis and monitoring of the intracellular calcium concentration suggest that PGE_1 induces smooth muscle relaxation by an inhibition of voltage-dependent calcium channels and a reduction in intracellular calcium concentration.[105] Clearly, relaxation is produced via a number of mechanisms.

That PGI_2 is unlikely to be a relaxant mediator was further supported by the finding that intracavernosal injection of PGI_2 in monkeys in vivo, at a dose of 100–200 mg, didn't increase arterial blood flow and, indeed, the resultant smooth muscle contraction produced a large reduction in cavernosal compliance.[106] This is in contrast to the increased cavernosal arterial blood flow and cavernous smooth muscle relaxation with PGE_1 injection in monkeys in vivo;[106]

intracavernosal injection of PGE$_1$ also caused an increase in intra-cavernosal pressure in rats.[107] Thus, the role of the endogenous penile PGs in normal physiological erection and erectile dysfunction remains uncertain.[108] However, PGE$_1$ would appear to have an appropriate profile of action for an erectogen; it is therefore surprising that there remains a paucity of information on the ability of the human corpora cavernosa to produce PGE$_1$.[109] Nevertheless, cavernosal PGE$_1$ receptors have been demonstrated in a variety of species, including man, using a radioligand-binding technique.[110]

Neuropeptide Y

Neuropeptide Y (NPY) has been co-localised with noradrenaline in adrenergic postganglionic neurones and may participate in vasoconstriction.[111,112] It has been demonstrated in the penile vasculature and in the corpus cavernosum of several species.[113–115] Interestingly, it has also been co-localised with VIP in the cavernous tissue and helicine arteries of the monkey.[113] NPY has been found in high concentration in the human corpus cavernosum and has been thought to be involved in the control of erection.[114] Wespes et al studied the distribution of NPY-containing nerves in the human penis and found NPY to be present in the fibres of the adventitia of arterial and venous vessels and among smooth muscle cells.[116] Crowe et al speculated that NPY might contribute to veno-occlusion as it was found in the media of the deep dorsal vein of the penis.[117] It was suggested that NPY may play a role in detumescence; however, the experimental evidence supporting the notion that there is a contractile mechanism involving NPY is insufficient.[118]

Calcitonin gene-related peptide

Calcitonin gene-related peptide (CGRP) immunoreactivity is present in the nerves of the corpus cavernosum in a variety of species, including man.[119] CGRP acts as a potent vasodilator in a variety of human blood vessels in vitro and is believed to act via an endothelium-dependent mechanism.[120] In the bull, the penile artery is relaxed via a direct action on the smooth muscle cells.[121]

27

Whereas one may speculate that high ET concentrations significantly contribute to both physiological flaccidity and erectile dysfunction and the role of the ETs remains to be fully established, they nevertheless constitute another component of the complex control mechanism of corporeal smooth muscle tone. In this context, it is interesting that increased ET binding was reported in a diabetic rabbit model.[138]

The role of second messengers

Corporeal smooth muscle tone is the most important factor determining the state of penile tumescence. The mechanisms influencing penile smooth muscle tone have their effects via complex intracellular second messenger systems.[9] The most important of these are cAMP, cGMP, calcium, potassium and inositol trisphosphate.

Cyclic AMP and cGMP were discovered more than 30 years ago and in the last 10 years much has been learned about receptor–cyclic nucleotide interactions and how GTP-binding proteins couple cAMP synthesis to receptor occupation. NO stimulates cGMP synthesis via soluble guanylate cyclase and cAMP is synthesised via the stimulation of adenylate cyclase by molecules such as PGE_1 and VIP. The intracellular levels of cyclic nucleotides are controlled by their synthesis, as well as their degradation by specific PDEs. The importance of the PDEs in the control of cyclic nucleotide levels has been realised for a number of years, but it is only recently that definitive work on their structure, function and regulation has been performed. It has become clear that different isozymes catalyse the synthetic and degradative processes and that more than one isozyme of adenylate cyclase can act as a catalyst. Furthermore, many different receptors can couple with cyclases with differing effects and end results – a wide variety of different mechanisms for controlling cAMP synthesis in a cell can now be visualised.

Intracellular calcium concentration and bioavailability are among the most important determinants in the control of smooth muscle tone. Free intracellular calcium results in the events of contraction-coupling; therefore, anything that will free this ion from intracellular stores will result in contraction. Membrane-active compounds which increase calcium concentration will increase tone and lead to penile flaccidity, whereas those which extrude calcium ions and therefore lead to a decrease of calcium concentration will decrease muscle tone and therefore lead to penile erection.

The importance of potassium channels in smooth muscle relaxation has only been recognised relatively recently.[139,140] There is now evidence that potassium channel openers relax vascular, tracheal and urinary bladder smooth muscle cells. This is accomplished by the opening of 86Rb-permeable potassium channels and the subsequent hyperpolarisation of the cells, which in turn leads to muscle relaxation by preventing the opening of voltage-dependent calcium channels.[141,142] The mechanisms that regulate corporeal smooth muscle tone are summarised in Fig. 2.6.

The role of sex hormones

Androgens, and testosterone in particular, are necessary (although not sufficient) for the maintenance of libido in men.[143] The relationships between androgen levels, libido and erectile function are incompletely understood. Similarly, the peripheral effects of androgens on the erectile tissues are not fully understood. Work on castrated dogs in vivo suggested that the androgen deficiency so produced had direct effects on the functioning of erectile tissues.[144] In a study using human tissues in an in vitro preparation, testosterone was without significant effect on contraction or relaxation.[145] Interestingly, in castrated rabbits NANC-mediated relaxation of erectile tissues was enhanced, although it was thought that the responsiveness to NO was not altered in this preparation.[146,147] It was noted that an observed reduction of noradrenaline release from adrenergic nerves might be the mechanism underpinning the changes.[147] In a rat study it was shown that castration reduced the erectile responses and that this was reversible by testosterone; the authors concluded that the effect of testosterone is to enhance the erectile response to cavernous nerve stimulation at a site peripheral to the spinal cord, and more specifically that it is the postganglionic

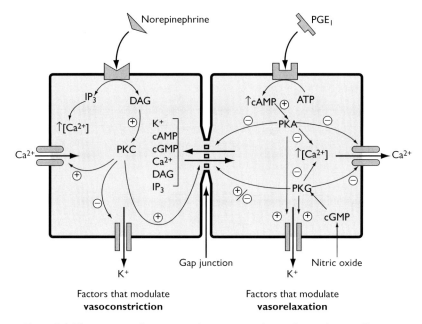

Figure 2.6 *The major mechanisms regulating corporeal smooth muscle tone. Shown are two corporal smooth muscle cells, interconnected by a gap junction at their lateral border. The left cell depicts the series of intracellular events linked to corporeal smooth muscle contraction – an elevation of intracellular calcium levels. The cell on the right depicts the events linked to corporeal smooth muscle relaxation – a diminution of transmembrane calcium flux, sequestration of intracellular calcium, membrane hyperpolarisation and, hence, smooth muscle relaxation. The effects of PKA, PKC and PKG on gap junctions, potassium and calcium channels are probably mediated by phosphorylation of specific amino acid residues on target proteins. PIP$_2$, phosphatidyl inositol; DAG, diacylglycerol; PKA, protein kinase A; PKG, protein kinase G. Reproduced with permission.*[181]

parasympathetic neurones that are the target for androgen action.[148] The roles of testosterone and prolactin in human sexual function were assessed in a study which suggested that both sexual behaviour and nocturnal erections were androgen-dependent, but that different thresholds of serum testosterone concentration applied to these different aspects of sexual function.[149]

Summary

Normal penile erection is a complex, multifactorial event dependent on the integrated functioning of a number of different elements. It is principally a haemodynamic event mediated via precise neural control mechanisms. The elements required for penile erection have been reviewed; the central role of NO, second messengers and smooth muscle relaxation within this process should be clearly appreciated. The release of nitric oxide of endothelial and neuronal origin results in the generation of cGMP via its activation of guanylate cyclase. The cGMP thus synthesised acts to alter intracellular calcium concentration and thus brings about penile smooth muscle relaxation and therefore erection (Fig. 2.7).

Aetiology of erectile dysfunction

For much of this century it was thought that erectile dysfunction was predominantly psychogenic in origin; over the past three decades it has been recognised that there are a large number of organic causes of erectile dysfunction. In a study of men over 70 with erectile dysfunction it was estimated that 80% of cases were actually due to organic causes.[150] It is important to remember that patients with an obvious organic cause for their erectile dysfunction may nevertheless have a considerable psychological component, and vice versa; indeed, to categorise patients as having either pure psychogenic or organic erectile dysfunction may be spurious.

There are many causes of organic erectile dysfunction (Table 2.1) and an ever-increasing number of drugs have also been implicated in the pathoaetiology of erectile dysfunction (see Table 4.3, Chapter 4). Physical disease may affect sexual function and erectile capacity in a number of ways. It may have direct effects by interfering with the substrates necessary for erection, e.g. by producing a vascular or neurological deficit, but the nonspecific effects of disease such as pain and fatigue may also contribute to sexual dysfunction.

Physical illness may also result in significant secondary psychological effects, such as loss of self-esteem and depression. Furthermore, there may be concern about the effects of sexual activity on health (e.g. in men with a history of ischaemic heart disease or recent myocardial infarction).

33

Finally, the effects of treatment itself may compromise the sexual and erectile functions of the individual: as already mentioned, many drugs are implicated in the pathogenesis of erectile dysfunction and may have their effects via a number of different mechanisms. A large number of surgical procedures, such as pelvic surgery or prostatectomy, may directly produce erectile dysfunction. Other procedures, such as colostomy, may produce a physical disfigurement, which results in a psychological component contributing to erectile dysfunction. In considering the pathogenesis of erectile failure, it is apparent that abnormalities in isolation or in combination can result in erectile dysfunction.

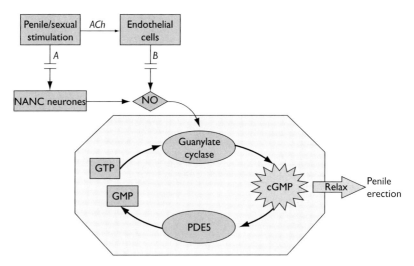

Figure 2.7 *Pathophysiology of erectile dysfunction in diabetes. Diagrammatic representation of pathways leading to and within a corpus cavernosal smooth muscle cell. In diabetes there are defects in nitric oxide smooth muscle relaxation due to neuropathy of the NANC fibres (A) and endothelial dysfunction (B). ACh, acetylcholine; cGMP, cyclic guanosine monophosphate; GTP, guanosine triphosphate; NANC, nonadrenergic-noncholinergic; NO, nitric oxide; PDE5, phosphodiesterase V.*

The aetiology of erectile dysfunction in diabetes mellitus

Erectile dysfunction occurs more commonly in men with diabetes mellitus than in the general population and, as in the non-diabetic

Table 2.1 Conditions associated with erectile dysfunction

Psychological disorders
- Anxiety about sexual performance
- Psychological trauma or abuse
- Misconceptions
- Sexual problems in the partner
- Depression
- Psychoses

Vascular disorders
- Peripheral vascular disease
- Hypertension
- Venous leak
- Pelvic trauma

Neurological disorders
- Stroke
- Multiple sclerosis
- Brain and spinal tumours
- Autonomic and peripheral neuropathies

Endocrine and metabolic disorders
- Diabetes
- Hypogonadism
- Hyperprolactinaemia
- Hypopituitarism
- Thyroid dysfunction
- Hyperlipidaemia
- Renal disease
- Liver disease

Structural abnormalities of the penis
- Penile curvature
- Hypospadias
- Micropenis
- Peyronie's disease
- Penile fibrosis
- Phimosis

Miscellaneous
- Surgery and trauma
- Smoking
- Drug and alcohol abuse

population, is probably due to a combination of physiological and psychological factors, as discussed in Chapter 3.[151,152] Diabetic men are not immune from psychogenic problems; indeed Jensen reported that many diabetic men have a marked superimposed psychological component.[153] There is little doubt, however, that in diabetes erectile dysfunction is particularly associated with neuropathy and vascular disease. In the recent past there has been debate as to the relative contribution of neuropathy and vascular disease. The vascular component may be due to both small and large vessel disease as well as microangiopathy. Furthermore, diabetes mellitus has wide-ranging effects on vasodilator mechanisms and causes endothelial dysfunction, the importance of which is now being increasingly recognised.[154] In addition, diabetic patients often have disturbances of lipid metabolism and may have hyperlipidaemia. Furthermore, there are significant abnormalities in receptor function as well as alterations in the normal transduction mechanisms required for penile smooth muscle relaxation.

The diabetic neuropathic process affects both the autonomic and peripheral nervous systems; however, it seems to preferentially affect the long parasympathetic fibres first (such as those responsible for the mediation of penile erection). We have previously discussed the changes observed in penile VIPergic innervation in both experimental and human diabetes.[155] Furthermore, dysfunctional cholinergic and adrenergic innervation has also been described in diabetes.[155,156]

There have been a number of studies that have attempted to determine the relative contributions of angiopathy and neuropathy to diabetic erectile dysfunction. The results of these investigations are somewhat at variance with each other. Some workers have stressed the importance and predominance of the neurological factor,[156,157] whereas others have stressed the importance of the angiopathic processes.[158,159] It seems that erectile dysfunction affecting the younger diabetic is usually due to a neuropathy, in contrast to older diabetics who may have a predominant vascular cause.[158] It is important to remember that there may also be a considerable psychogenic component, not least as a result of the chronic nature of the disease.[158,160] Furthermore, diabetes also has deleterious effects on endothelial function as well as corporeal smooth muscle relaxation: it has been elegantly demonstrated that diabetes impairs neurogenic and endothelium-dependent relaxation of rabbit and human penile smooth muscle.[23,161] Diabetes was shown to decrease PGI_2 synthesis in streptozotocin-diabetic rats.[162] More recently it has been shown that the density of endothelin binding to rat corpus cavernosum is also significantly increased in streptozotocin-induced diabetes mellitus; clearly this may contribute to diabetic erectile dysfunction and is further evidence of the global abnormalities of endothelial dysfunction seen in diabetes.[138]

The role of diabetic neuropathy

Neuropathy (clinical or subclinical) probably affects over one-third of patients with diabetes mellitus. The pathophysiology of diabetic neuropathy is complex and recent advances in our understanding have opened the door for newer therapeutic approaches. The mechanisms responsible are a combination of metabolic and microvascular alterations that result in both structural and functional abnormalities. The microvascular mechanism is essentially the small vessels that supply the neurones, the vasa nervorum, being affected by atherosclerosis and resulting in hypoxia with obvious subsequent functional changes. Small vessel disease may be a key mechanism for neuropathy and, indeed, microscopically the vasa nervorum of these patients are occluded.[163]

Vasculogenic erectile dysfunction

Erectile dysfunction may also be the result of a lack of arterial supply due to occlusive vascular disease (arteriogenic impotence), or to the inability of the penis to trap blood by the veno-occlusive mechanism (venous leak), or a combination of both. Atherosclerosis may result in narrowing of the penile and/or pelvic vessels, vascular damage to the erectile and endothelial tissues, and a secondary venous leak. Erectile dysfunction due to occlusive vascular disease may therefore be associated with conditions such as diabetes mellitus, ischaemic heart disease, hypertension, peripheral vascular disease and hyperlipidaemia. This has been substantiated in a number of studies linking vascular risk factors with erectile dysfunction.[151,164,165]

The importance of endothelial dysfunction and the nitric oxide pathway in the pathophysiology of impotence in diabetes

Diabetes is characterised by an 'endotheliopathy' which may be intrinsic to the insulin-resistant state and may even antedate the onset of type II diabetes.[155] As described above, both endothelium-derived and neuronal nitric oxide play a crucial role in the process of penile erection. The crucial study which lay the groundwork to our present understanding of the pathophysiology of impotence in diabetes was that of Saenz deTejada and colleagues in 1989.[23] Samples of cavernosal tissue were taken from 21 diabetic and 42 non-diabetic men undergoing implant operations. Smooth muscle contraction was induced by noradrenaline and relaxation with electrical field stimulation. The effects of acetylcholine, which generates endothelial NO, and sodium nitroprusside, an NO donor, were studied. The results suggested that tumescence is produced as a result of direct NO release from nerve terminals and from NO released from endothelial cells mediated by acetylcholine. In the diabetic subjects both pathways were impaired compared with non-diabetics. In other words, impotence in diabetes may be due to a failure of NO-mediated smooth muscle relaxation due to both autonomic neuropathy and endothelial cell dysfunction (Fig. 2.7). Further powerful evidence of the central role of the nitric oxide pathway in the aetiopathogenesis of erectile dysfunction comes from the efficacy of phosphodiesterase inhibitors in treating impotence (see Chapter 4).

Erectile dysfunction as a marker of cardiovascular risk

Further evidence of the role of endothelial dysfunction in the aetiology of ED is provided by the strong association between (ED) and cardiovascular disease erectile dysfunction.[166] This may be because they share common risk factors but is more likely because they are both manifestations of endothelial dysfunction. The endothelium has endocrine and paracrine functions and one of its most important products is nitric oxide (NO) which possesses potent anti-atherogenic properties, inhibits platelet aggregation and regulates vascular tone.[167] As described above, NO derived from both nerve terminals and the vascular endothelium has a central role in the physiology of erection.

There are, therefore, theoretical reasons to believe that the ED might be an early marker of endothelial dysfunction and a risk factor for cardiovascular disease. Evidence to support this comes from a small study of endothelial function in impotent men. Endothelial function, as assessed by measuring arterial pulse wave velocity during reactive hyperaemia, was abnormal in the diabetic men both with and without ED and, interestingly, highly abnormal in the non-diabetic men who were healthy apart from the presence of ED.[168] This small study would suggest the most men who present with ED already have marked endothelial dysfunction. The implications of this are interesting. It may be that ED is one of the earliest markers of endothelial dysfunction and an important marker of cardiovascular risk.

Other factors

Hypertension

Hypertension is a risk factor for erectile dysfunction[151,165,166] and up to 45% of diabetic men are hypertensive. Unfortunately, the treatment of hypertension is often itself complicated by erectile dysfunction. Antihypertensive drugs may have either central or peripheral effects, or both, e.g. beta blockers. However, there is evidence that hypertension by itself may be a cause of erectile dysfunction. Nevertheless, as a general principle it is usually good practice to evaluate the presence of erectile dysfunction before prescribing for hypertension; if it is already present, then patients should be carefully counselled that it might be made worse. Unfortunately, attempts to modify antihypertensive medication to improve the erectile dysfunction do not usually meet with success.

Failure of the veno-occlusive mechanism

Venous outflow restriction is an essential requirement for the initiation and maintenance of penile erection.[71] A failure of the penis to trap blood has been termed 'venous leak'; such an inability to trap arterial blood within the penis is a frequent abnormality seen in erectile dysfunction. It has been estimated that up to 30% of men suffering with erectile dysfunction will have venous incompetence as a contributing cause for their impotence.[170] Despite the available evidence, the precise mechanism of veno-occlusion remains somewhat controversial, and therefore it is not surprising that the exact cause of venous leakage remains unknown. However, venous leakage increasingly appears to result primarily from alterations of intracorporeal structures and the term veno-corporeal incompetence is preferable to venous leak.[171]

Medication-induced erectile dysfunction

Many drugs have been implicated in the aetiology of erectile dysfunction (Table 4.3, Chapter 4). However, drug-related effects may sometimes be difficult to separate from the effects of chronic disease. Drugs may affect erectile performance at a number of levels, including central, peripheral and target organ. Antihypertensive agents are the most commonly cited drugs in causing erectile dysfunction. Hypertension is common, and as a result antihypertensives are probably the most frequently used drugs in medical practice. As alluded to previously, beta blockers have their effects centrally, where they act to lower libido; peripherally, by reducing the penile perfusion pressure; and at the endothelial level, by causing decreased PG production.[52,172,173] The thiazide diuretics cause erectile dysfunction in some 9% of patients who take them.[174] The drugs that have the lowest incidence of erectile dysfunction as a side effect of the treatment of hypertension are calcium channel blockers, angiotensin converting enzyme (ACE) inhibitors and, in particular, the alpha blockers.[175,176] The major tranquillisers, the phenothiazines, monoamine oxidase inhibitors and the tricyclic antidepressants are all commonly used. The sedation that they produce as well as their anticholinergic and sympatholytic effects are thought to be the responsible factors. The phenothiazines can also raise prolactin levels that can interfere with luteinising hormone and testosterone secretion.

Renal failure

Diabetes mellitus is a major cause of chronic renal failure, which is a well-documented cause of erectile dysfunction; it is present in between 38 and 80% of dialysis patients, some 20–55% being completely impotent.[177] The condition is often exacerbated after the beginning of dialysis and of those men who have a renal transplant, 10% will have post-surgical erectile dysfunction; this figure rises to 30% after a second transplant.[178]

Neurogenic erectile dysfunction

The commonest peripheral nervous system causes of erectile dysfunction are those seen in diabetic neuropathy, which can affect both the autonomic and somatic fibres. However, a number of other processes can result in neurogenic dysfunction. Cord compression from a prolapsed intervertebral disc or cauda equina tumours can result in erectile dysfunction. A common iatrogenic cause of nerve damage is that due to radical pelvic surgery where the cavernous nerves are particularly at risk. In this context the recent advances such as the development of the technique of nerve-sparing radical prostatectomy have apparently reduced the incidence of erectile dysfunction associated with such procedures.[21]

Smoking and erectile dysfunction

Smoking has been clearly linked to erectile dysfunction as a risk factor for its development.[151,165] Experimental data have implicated disturbances of prostaglandin metabolism in the aetiology of erectile failure: for example, rats that have been rendered diabetic have decreased penile PGI_2 synthesis[162] and, similarly, cigarette smoke extracts (and not nicotine) inhibit PGI_2 production in rat penile tissue.[179] It may be that an interference with penile prostaglandin metabolism may account, at least in part, for the impotence that is associated with certain drugs.

Notwithstanding the effects on prostaglandin synthesis, smoking has been demonstrated to affect the contractile activity of penile arteries, and data support the notion that smoking may further compromise penile physiology in men who are experiencing difficulty in maintaining erections long enough for satisfactory intercourse.[180] Smoking may act as a risk factor for erectile dysfunction by reducing high-density lipoprotein (HDL) and increasing fibrinogen levels. Low HDL was a predictor of erectile dysfunction in the Massachusetts Male Aging and Cooper Clinic (Dallas) studies;[151,181] furthermore, both elevated fibrinogen and reduced HDL concentrations are known predictors of ischaemic heart disease.

Summary

The pathophysiology of erectile dysfunction in men with diabetes is clearly a multifactorial phenomenon; many investigators have reported multiple deficits in the mechanisms that underpin normal erectile activity. Diabetes mellitus exerts its powerful effects via a combination of psychological, neuropathic, angiopathic and metabolic mechanisms, but perhaps of central importance are the effects of autonomic neuropathy and endothelial and vascular dysfunction, leading to a failure of nitric oxide-mediated smooth muscle relaxation.

References

1. Newman HF, Northup JD. Mechanism of human penile erection: an overview. Urology 1981; 17:399–408.
2. Aboseif SR, Lue TF. Haemodynamics of penile erection. Urol Clin North Am 1988; 15:1–7.
3. Luangkhot R, Rutchik S, Agarwal V et al. Collagen alterations in the corpus cavernosum of men with sexual dysfunction. J Urol 1992; 148:467–71.
4. Krane SM, Neer RM, Smith Jr LH, Thier SO, eds. Pathophysiology: The Biological Principles of Disease, 2nd edn. Philadelphia: W.B. Saunders; 1985: 611.
5. Bossart MI, Spjut JJ, Scott FB. Ultrastructural analysis of human penile corpus cavernosum: its significance in tumescence and detumescence. Urology 1980; 15:448–56.
6. Conti G, Virag R. Human penile erection and organic impotence: normal histology and histopathology. Urol Int 1989; 44(5):303–8.
7. Heaton JP. Synthetic nitrovasodilators are effective, in vitro, in relaxing penile tissue from impotent men: the findings and their implications. Can J Physiol Pharmacol 1989; 67:78–81.
8. Campos de Carvalho AC, Moreno AP, Christ G, et al. Gap junctions between human corpus cavernosum smooth muscle cells: identity of the connexin type and unitary conductance events. J Cell Biol 1990; 111:153a, 835.

9. Christ GJ, Moreno A, Parker ME et al. Intercellular communication through gap junctions: a potential role in pharmacomechanical coupling and syncytial tissue contraction in vascular smooth muscle isolated from the human corpus cavernosum. Life Sci 1991; 49:PL195–200.

10. Moreno AP, Campos de Carvalho AC, Christ GJ et al. Gap junctions between human corpus cavernosum smooth muscle cells in primary culture: electrophysiological and biochemical characteristics. Int J Impot Res 1990; 2 (suppl) 2–55.

11. Breza J, Aboseif SR, Orvis BR et al. Detailed anatomy of penile neuro-vascular structures: surgical significance. Urology 1989; 141:437–43.

12. Valji K, Bookstein JJ. Transluminal angioplasty in the treatment of arterio-genic impotence. Cardiovasc Intervent Radiol 1988; 11:245–52.

13. Bahren W, Gall H, Scherb W et al. Arterial anatomy and arteriographic diagnosis of arteriogenic impotence. Cardiovasc Intervent Radiol 1988; 11:195–210.

14. Flanigan DP, Sobinsky KR, Schuler JJ et al. Internal iliac artery revascu-larisation in the treatment of vasculogenic impotence. Arch Surg 1985; 120:271–4.

15. Bookstein JJ. Penile angiography: the last angiographic frontier. Am J Radiol 1988; 150:47–54.

16. Lue TF, Tanagho EA. Tanagho EA, Lue TF, McClure RD, eds. Contem-porary Management of Impotence and Infertility. Baltimore: Williams and Wilkins, 1988: 39.

17. Andersson KE, Wagner G. Physiology of penile erection. Physiol Rev 1995; 75 (1):191–235.

18. Weiss HD. The physiology of human penile erection. Ann Intern Med 1972; 76:793–9.

19. Nunez R, Gross GH, Sachs BD. Origin and central projections of rat dorsal penile nerve: possible direct projection to autonomic and somatic neurons by primary afferents of nonmuscle origin. J Comp Neurol 1986; 247:417–29.

20. Steers WD, Mallory B, De Groat WC. Electrophysiological analysis of penile reflexes in the rat. Am J Physiol 1988; 254:R989–1000.

21. Walsh PC, Donker PJ. Impotence following radical prostatectomy: insight into etiology and prevention. J Urol 1982; 130:1237–41.

22. Lepor H, Gregerman M, Crosby R et al. Precise localization of the autonomic nerves from the pelvic plexus to the corpora cavernosa: a detailed anatomical study of the adult male pelvis. J Urol 1985; 133:207–12.

23. Saenz deTejada IS, Goldstein II, Azadzoi K et al. Impaired neurogenic and endothelium-mediated relaxation of penile smooth muscle from diabetic men with impotence. N Engl J Med 1989; 320:1025–30.

24. De Groat WC, Booth AM. Physiology of male sexual function. Ann Intern Med 1980; 92:329–40.

25. Saenz deTejada I, Goldstein I, Blanco R et al. Smooth muscle of the corpora cavernosae: role in penile erection. Surg Forum 1985; 36:623–4.
26. Fournier GR Jr, Juenemann KP, Lue TF, Tanagho EA. Mechanism of venous occlusion during canine penile erection: an anatomic demonstration. J Urol 1987; 137:163–7.
27. Wespes E, Schulman CC. Hemodynamic role of tunica albuginea during erection. Acta Urol Belg 1986; 54:114.
28. Furchgott RF, Zawadski JV. The obligatory role of endothelial cells in the relaxation of arterial smooth muscle cells by acetylcholine. Nature 1980; 288:373–6.
29. Furchgott RF. Studies on endothelium-dependent vasodilation and the endothelium-derived relaxing factor. Acta Physiol Scand 1990; 139:257–70.
30. Palmer RM, Ferrige AG, Moncada S. Nitric oxide release accounts for the biological activity of endothelium-derived relaxing factor. Nature 1987; 327:524–6.
31. Burnett AL, Lowenstein CJ, Bredt DS et al. Nitric oxide: a physiological mediator of penile erection. Science 1992; 257(5068):401–3.
32. Sjostrand NO, Klinge E. Principal mechanisms controlling penile retraction and protrusion in rabbits. Acta Physiol Scand 1979; 106:199–214.
33. Brindley GS. Pilot experiments on the actions of drugs injected into the human corpus cavernosum penis. Br J Pharmacol 1986; 87:495–500.
34. Brindley GS, Sauerwein D, Hendry WH. Hypogastric stimulators for obtaining semen from paraplegic men. Br J Urol 1989; 64:72–7.
35. Shirai M, Sasaki K, Rikimaru A. Histochemical investigation on the distribution of adrenergic and cholinergic nerves in human penis. Tohoku J Exp Med 1972; 107:403–4.
36. Benson GS, McConnell J, Lipshultz LI et al. Neuromorphology and neuropharmacology of the human penis: an in vitro study. J Clin Invest 1980; 65:506–13.
37. Gu J, Polak JM, Probert L et al. Peptidergic innervation of the human male genital tract. J Urol 1983; 130:386–91.
38. Hedlund H, Andersson KE, Mattiasson A. Pre- and postjunctional adreno- and muscarinic receptor functions in the isolated human corpus spongiosum urethrae. J Auton Pharmacol 1984; 4:241–9.
39. Adaikan PG, Karim SM. Adrenoceptors in the human penis. J Auton Pharmacol 1981; 1:199–203.
40. McConnell J, Benson GS. Innervation of human penile blood vessels. Neurourol Urodyn 1982; 1:199–210.
41. Hedlund H, Andersson KE. Comparison of the responses to drugs acting on adrenoceptors and muscarinic receptors in human isolated corpus cavernosum and cavernous artery. J Auton Pharmacol 1985; 5:81–8.
42. Kimura K, Kawanishi Y, Tamura M, Imagawa A. Assessment of the alpha-adrenergic receptors in isolated human and canine corpus cavernosum tissue. Int J Impot Res 1989; 1:185–9.

43. Christ GJ, Maayani S, Valcic M, Melman A. Pharmacological studies of human erectile tissue: characteristics of spontaneous contractions and alterations in α-adrenoceptor responsiveness with age and disease in isolated tissues. Br J Pharmacol 1990; 101:375–81.

44. Saenz deTejada I, Kim N, Lagan I et al. Regulation of adrenergic activity in penile corpus cavernosum. J Urol 1989; 142:1117–21.

45. Kirkeby HJ, Forman A, Sorensen S, Andersson KE. Alpha-adrenoceptor function in isolated penile circumflex veins from potent and impotent men. J Urol 1989; 142:1369–71.

46. Fontaine J, Schulman CC, Wespes E. Postjunctional α1- and α2-like adrenoceptors in human isolated deep dorsal vein of the penis. Br J Pharmacol 1986; 89:493.

47. Price DT, Schwinn DA, Kim JH et al. Alpha adrenergic receptor subtype mRNA expression in human corpus cavernosum. J Urol 1993; 149:285A.

48. Brindley GS. Cavernosal alpha-blockade: a new technique for investigating and treating erectile impotence. Br J Psychiatry 1983; 143:332–7.

49. Brindley GS. A new treatment for priapism. Lancet 1984; 2:220–1.

50. De Meyer JM, De Sy WA. Intracavernous injection of noradrenaline to interrupt erections during surgical interventions. Eur Urol 1986; 12:169–70.

51. Azadoi KM, Payton T, Krane RJ, Goldstein I. Effects of intracavernosal trazodone hydrochloride: animal and human studies. J Urol 1990; 144:1277–82.

52. Andersson KE, Holmquist F, Wagner G. Pharmacology of drugs used for treatment of erectile dysfunction and priapism. Int J Impot Res 1991; 3:155–72.

53. Adaikan PG, Lau LC, Ng SC, Ratnam SS. Physio-pharmacology of human penile erection – autonomic/nitregic neurotransmission and receptors of the human corpus cavernosum. Asian Pac J Pharmacol 1991; 6:213–27.

54. Creed KE, Carati CJ, Adamson GM, Callahan SM. Responses of erectile tissue from impotent men to pharmacological agents. Br J Urol 1989; 64:180–2.

55. Eckhardt C. Untersuchungen über die Erection des Penis beim Hunde. Beitrage zur Anatomie und Physiologie 1863; 3:123–66.

56. Langley JN, Anderson HK. The innervation of the pelvic and adjoining viscera. Part III. The external generative organs. J Physiol (Lond) 1895; 19:85–121.

57. Nikolsky W. Ein Beitrag zur Physiologie der Nervi Erigentes. Arch Anat Physiol (Lpz) 1879; 209:221.

58. Klinge E, Sjostrand NO. Suppression of the excitatory adrenergic neurotransmission; a possible role of cholinergic nerves in the retractor penis muscle. Acta Physiol Scand 1977; 100:368–76.

59. Saenz deTejada I, Blanco R, Goldstein I et al. Cholinergic neurotransmission in human corpus cavernosum. I. Responses of isolated tissue. Am J Physiol 1988; 254:H459–H467.

60. Godec CJ, Bates H. Cholinergic receptors in corpora cavernosa. Investig Urol 1984; 24:31–3.
61. Blanco R, Saenz deTejada I, Goldstein I et al. Cholinergic neurotransmission in human corpus cavernosum. II. Acetylcholine synthesis. Am J Physiol 1988; 254:H468–H472.
62. Traish AM, Carson MP, Kim N et al. Characterization of muscarinic acetylcholine receptors in human penile corpus cavernosum: studies on whole tissue and cultured endothelium. J Urol 1990; 144:1036–40.
63. Adaikan PG, Karim SM, Kottegoda SR, Ratnam SS. Cholinoreceptors in the corpus cavernosum muscle of the human penis. J Auton Pharmacol 1983; 3:107–11.
64. Andersson KE, Hedlund W, Mattiasson A et al. Relaxation of isolated corpus spongiosum induced by vasoactive intestinal polypeptide, substance P, carbachol and electrical field stimulation. World J Urol 1983; 1:203–8.
65. Andersson PO, Bloom SR, Mellander S. Haemodynamics of pelvic nerve induced penile erection in the dog: possible mediation by vasoactive intestinal polypeptide. J Physiol (Lond) 1984; 350:209–24.
66. Larsson B, Andersson KE, Mattiasson A. Influence of antimuscarinics on alpha-adrenoceptors in the female rabbit urethra. Act Physiol Scand 1984; 120:537–42.
67. Stief CG, Benard F, Bosch RJLH et al. Acetylcholine as a possible neurotransmitter in penile erection. J Urol 1989; 14:1444–8.
68. Wagner G, Brindley GS. Zorgniotti AW, Rossi G, eds. Vasculogenic Impotence. Springfield, Illinois: Thomas, 1980: 77–81.
69. Trigo-Rocha F, Hsu GL, Donatucci CF, Lue TF. The role of cyclic adenosine monophosphate, cyclic guanosine monophosphate, endothelium and nonadrenergic, noncholinergic neurotransmission in canine penile erection. J Urol 1993; 149:872–7.
70. Lowenstein CJ, Dinerman JL, Snyder SH. Nitric oxide: a physiologic messenger. Ann Intern Med 1994; 120:227–37.
71. Saenz deTejada I, Goldstein I, Krane RJ. Local control of penile erection. Nerves, smooth muscle and endothelium. Urol Clin North Am 1988; 15:9–15.
72. Burnstock G. Regulation of local blood flow by neurohumoral substances released from perivascular nerves and endothelial cells. Acta Physiol Scand 1988; 133(571):53–9.
73. Keast JR. A possible neural source of nitric oxide in the rat penis. Neurosci Lett 1992; 143:69–73.
74. Bush PA, Aronson WJ, Buga GM et al. Nitric oxide is a potent relaxant of human and rabbit corpus cavernosum. J Urol 1992; 147:1650–5.
75. Rajfer J, Aronson WJ, Bush PA et al. Nitric oxide as a mediator of relaxation of the corpus cavernosum in response to nonadrenergic, noncholinergic neurotransmission. N Engl J Med 1992; 326:90–4.

76. Holmquist F, Hedlund H, Andersson KE. l-N^G-nitroarginine inhibits non-adrenergic, non-cholinergic relaxation of human isolated corpus cavernosum. Acta Physiol Scand 1991; 141:441–2.

77. Ignarro LJ, Bush PA, Buga GM et al. Nitric oxide and cyclic GMP formation upon electrical field stimulation cause relaxation of corpus cavernosum smooth muscle. Biochem Biophys Res Commun 1990; 170(2):843–50.

78. Kim N, Azadzoi KM, Goldstein I, Saenz deTejada I. A nitric oxide-like factor mediates nonadrenergic-noncholinergic neurogenic relaxation of penile corpus cavernosum smooth muscle. J Clin Invest 1991; 88:112–18.

79. Knispel HH, Goessl C, Beckman R. Nitric oxide mediates relaxation in rabbit and human corpus cavernosum smooth muscle. Urol Res 1992; 20:253–7.

80. Burnett AL, Tillman SL, Chang TSK et al. Immunohistochemical localization of nitric oxide synthase in the autonomic innervation of the human penis. J Urol 1993; 150:73–6.

81. Bush PA, Aronson WJ, Rajfer J et al. Comparison of nonadrenergic, noncholinergic and nitric oxide-mediated relaxation of corpus cavernosum. Int J Impot Res 1992; 4:85–93.

82. Holmquist F, Andersson KE, Hedlund H. Characterization of inhibitory neurotransmission in the isolated corpus cavernosum from rabbit and man. J Physiol (Lond) 1992; 449:295–311.

83. Holmquist F, Fridstand M, Hedlund H, Andersson KE. Actions of 3-morpholinosydnonimin (SIN-1) on rabbit isolated penile erectile tissue. J Urol 1993; 150:1310–15.

84. Kim N, Vardi Y, Padma-Nathan H, et al. Oxygen tension regulates erection by modulating nitric oxide production in corpus cavernosum. Int J Impot Res 1992; (4, Suppl 2):A3.

85. Kim N, Vardi Y, Padma-Nathan H et al. Oxygen tension regulates the nitric oxide pathway. J Clin Invest 1993; 91:437–42.

86. Huang PL, Dawson TM, Bredt DS et al. Targeted disruption of the neuronal nitric oxide synthase gene. Cell 1993; 75:1273–86.

87. Said SI. Bloom SR, Polak JM, eds. Gut Hormones. 2nd edn. Edinburgh: Churchill Livingstone; 1981: 379–84.

88. Ganz P, Sandrock AW, Landis SC et al. Vasoactive intestinal peptide: vasodilatation and cyclic AMP generation. Am J Physiol 1986; 250:H755–60.

89. Chakder S, Rattan S. Involvement of cAMP and cGMP in relaxation of internal anal sphincter by neural stimulation, VIP, and NO. Am J Physiol 1993; 264(4pt1):G702–7.

90. Grider JR, Murthy KS, Jin J-G, Makhlouf GM. Stimulation of nitric oxide from muscle cells by VIP: prejunctional enhancement of VIP release. Am J Physiol 1992; 262(4pt1):G774–8.

91. Kinsey AC, Pomeroy W, Martin CE, Kinsey AC, Pomeroy W, Martin CE, eds. Sexual Behaviour in the Human Man. Philadelphia: WB Saunders, 1948: 218–62.

92. Polak JM, Mina S, Gu J, Bloom SR. Vipergic nerves in the penis. Lancet 1981; 2:217–19.

93. Kirkeby HJ, Fahrenkrug J, Holmquist F, Ottesen B. Vasoactive intestinal polypeptide (VIP) and peptide histidine methionine (PHM) in human penile corpus cavernosum tissue and circumflex veins: localization and in vitro effects. Eur J Clin Invest 1992; 22:24–30.

94. Pickard RS, Powell PH, Zar MA. Evidence against vasoactive intestinal polypeptide as the relaxant neurotransmitter in human cavernosal smooth muscle. Br J Pharmacol 1993; 108:497–500.

95. Kiely EA, Bloom SR, Williams G. Penile response to intracavernosal vasoactive intestinal polypeptide alone and in combination with other vasoactive agents. Br J Urol 1989; 64:191–4.

96. Feldman HA, McKinlay JB, Watertown MA et al. Erectile dysfunction. Cardiovascular disease, and cardiovascular risk factors. Prospective results in a large sample of Massachusetts men. J Urol 1998; 159(suppl):91.

97. Roy AC, Tan SM, Kottegoda SR, Ratnam SS. Ability of the human corpora cavernosa muscle to generate prostaglandins and thromboxanes in vitro. IRCS J Med Sci 1984; 12:608–9.

98. Roy AC, Adaikan PG, Sen DK, Ratnam SS. Prostaglandin 15-hydroxyde-hydrogenase activity in human penile corpora cavernosa and its significance in prostaglandin-mediated erection. Br J Urol 1989; 64:180–2.

99. Jeremy JY, Morgan RJ, Mikhailidis DP, Dandona P. Prostacyclin synthesis by the corpora cavernosa of the human penis: evidence for muscarinic control and pathological implications. Prostaglandins Leukot Med 1986; 23:211–16.

100. Klinge E, Sjostrand NO. Comparative study of some isolated mammalian smooth muscle effectors of penile erection. Acta Physiol Scand 1977; 100:354–67.

101. Hedlund H, Andersson KE. Contraction and relaxation induced by some prostanoids in isolated human penile erectile tissue and cavernous artery. J Urol 1985; 134:1245–50.

102. Mellion BT, Ignarro LJ, Myers CB et al. Inhibition of human platelet aggregation by S-nitrosothiols. Heme-dependent activation of soluble guanylate cyclase and stimulation of cyclic GMP activation. Mol Pharmacol 1983; 23(3):653–64.

103. Molderings GJ, Gothert M, Van Ahlen H, Porst H. Norarenaline release in human corpus cavernosum and its modulation via presynaptic alpha$_2$-adrenoceptors. Fundam Clin Pharmacol 1989; 102:261–7.

104. Bhargava G, Valcic M, Melman A. Human corpora cavernosa smooth muscle cells in culture: influence of catecholamines and prostaglandins on cAMP formation. Int J Impot Res 1990; 2 (Suppl 2):35–6.

105. Derouet H, Eckert R, Trautwein W, Ziegler M. Muscular cavernous single cell analysis in patients with venoocclusive dysfunction. Eur Urol 1994; 25:145–50.

106. Bosch RJLH, Benard F, Aboseif SR. Changes in penile hemodynamics after intracavernous injection of prostaglandin E_1 and prostaglandin I_2 in pig-tailed monkeys. Int J Impot Res 1989; 1:211–21.

107. Chen KK, Chan JY, Chang LS et al. Intracavernous pressure as an experimental index in a rat model for the evaluation of penile erection. J Urol 1992; 147:1124–8.

108. Miller MAW, Morgan RJ. Eicosanoids, erections and erectile dysfunction. Prostaglandins Leukot Essent Fatty Acids 1994; 51(1):1–9.

109. Mikhailidis DP, Jeremy JY, Shoukry K, Virag R. Eicosanoids, impotence and pharmacologically induced erection. Prostaglandins Leukot Essent Fatty Acids 1990; 40:239–42.

110. Aboseif S, Riemer RK, Stackl W et al. Quantification of prostaglandin E1 receptors in cavernous tissue of men, monkeys and dogs. Urol Int 1993; 50:148–52.

111. Grundemar L, Hakansson R. Multiple neuropeptide Y receptors are involved in cardiovascular regulation. Peripheral and central mechanisms. Gen Pharmacol 1993; 24:785–96.

112. Wahlestedt C, Reis DJ. Neuropeptide Y-related peptides and their receptors – are the receptors potential therapeutic drug targets? Annu Rev Pharmacol Toxicol 1993; 32:309–52.

113. Schmalbruch H, Wagner G. Vasoactive intestinal polypeptide (VIP)- and neuropeptide Y (NPY)-containing nerves in the penile cavernous tissue of green monkeys (*Cercopithecus aethiops*). Cell Tissue Res 1989; 256:529–41.

114. Adrian TE, Gu J, Allen JM et al. Neuropeptide Y in the human male genital tract. Life Sci 1984; 35:2643–8.

115. Kirkeby HJ, Jorgensen J, Ottesen B. Neuropeptide Y (NPY) in human penile corpus cavernosum and circumflex veins. J Urol 1990; 145:605–9.

116. Wespes E, Schiffman S, Gilloteaux J et al. Study of neuropeptide Y-containing fibers in the human penis. Cell Tissue Res 1988; 254:69–74.

117. Crowe R, Burnstock G, Dickinson IK, Pryor JP. The human penis: an unusual penetration of NPY-immunoreactive nerves within the medial muscle coat of the deep dorsal vein. J Urol 1991; 145:1292–6.

118. Hedlund H, Andersson KE. Effects of some peptides on isolated human penile erectile tissue and cavernous artery. Acta Physiol Scand 1985; 124:413–19.

119. Stief CG, Wetterauer U, Schaebsdau FH, Jonas U. Calcitonin-gene-related peptide: a possible role in human penile erection and its therapeutic application in impotent patients. J Urol 1991; 146:1010–14.

120. Crossman D, McEwan J, Macdermot J et al. Human calcitonin-gene-related peptide activates adenylate cyclase and releases prostacyclin from human umbilical vein endothelial cells. Br J Pharmacol 1987; 92:695–701.

121. Alaranta S, Uusitalo H, Hautamaki AM, Klinge E. Calcitonin-gene-related peptide: immunohistochemical localization in, and effects on, the bovine penile artery. Int J Impot Res 1991; 3:49–59.

122. Stief CG, Benard F, Bosch R et al. Calcitonin-gene-related peptide: possibly neurotransmitter contributes to penile erection in monkeys. Urology 1993; 41:397–401.

123. Kaiser FE, Viosca SP, Morley JE et al. Impotence and aging: clinical and hormonal factors. J Am Geriat Soc 1988; 36:511–19.

124. Klinge E, Sjostrand NO. Contraction and relaxation of the retractor penis muscle and the penile artery of the bull. Acta Physiol Scand 1974; 420:1–88.

125. Keast JR, De Groat WC. Immunohistochemical characterization of pelvic neurons which project to the bladder, colon, or penis in rats. J Comp Neurol 1989; 288:387–400.

126. Keast JR, De Groat WC. Segmental distribution and peptide content of primary afferent neurons innervating the urogenital organs and colon of male rats. J Comp Neurol 1992; 319:615–23.

127. Pentilla O, Vartiainen A. Acetylcholine, histamine, 5-hydroxytryptamine and catecholamine contents of mammalian penile erectile tissue and urethral tissue. Acta Pharmacol Toxicol 1964; 21:145–51.

128. Sathananthan AH, Adaikan PG, Lau LC et al. Fine structure of the human corpus cavernosum. Arch Androl 1991; 26:107–17.

129. Ambache N, Killick SW, Aboo Zar M. Extraction from ox retractor penis of an inhibitory substance which mimicks its atropine-resistant neurogenic relaxation. Br J Pharmacol 1975; 54:409–10.

130. Klinge E. The effect of some substances on the isolated bull retractor penis muscle. Acta Physiol Scand 1970; 78:280–8.

131. Luduena FP, Grigas EO. Pharmacological study of autonomic innervation of dog retractor penis. Am J Physiol 1966; 210:435–44.

132. Adaikan PG, Karim SM. Effects of histamine on the human penis muscle in vitro. Eur J Pharmacol 1977; 45:261–5.

133. Kelm M, Feelisch M, Krebber T et al. Mechanisms of histamine-induced coronary vasodilatation: H1-receptor-mediated release of endothelium-derived nitric oxide. J Vasc Res 1993; 30:132–8.

134. Kirkeby HJ, Forman A, Sorensen S, Andersson KE. Effects of noradrenaline, 5-hydroxytryptamine and histamine on human penile cavernous tissue and circumflex veins. Int J Impot Res 1989; 1:181–8.

135. McGrath MA, Shepherd JT. Inhibition of adrenergic neurotransmission in canine vascular smooth muscle by histamine: mediation by H2-receptors. Circ Res 1976; 39:566–73.

136. Holmquist F, Kirkeby HJ, Larsson B et al. Functional effects, binding sites and immunolocalization of endothelin-1 in isolated penile tissues from man and rabbit. J Pharmacol Exp Ther 1992; 261:795–802.

137. Saenz deTejada I, Carson MP, de las Morenas A et al. Endothelin: localization, synthesis, activity, and receptor types in human penile corpus cavernosum. Am J Physiol 1991; 261:H1078–85.
138. Bell CRW, Sullivan ME, Dashwood MR et al. The density and distribution of endothelin-1 and endothelin receptor subtypes in normal and diabetic rat corpus cavernosum. Br J Urol 1995; 76:203–7.
139. Hamilton TC, Weston AH. Cromakalim and pinacidil: novel drugs which open potassium channels in smooth muscle. Gen Pharmacol 1989; 20:1–9.
140. Quast U, Cook NS. Moving together: K^+ channel openers and ATP-sensitive K^+ channels. Trends Pharmacol Sci 1989; 10:431–5.
141. Longman SD, Hamilton TC. Potassium channel activator drugs: mechanisms of action, pharmacological properties, and therapeutic potential. Med Res Rev 1992; 12:73–148.
142. Cook NS. The pharmacology of potassium channels and their therapeutic potential. Trends Pharmacol Sci 1988; 9:21–8.
143. Everitt BJ, Bancroft J. Of rats and men: the comparative approach to male sexuality. Annu Rev Sex Res 1991; 2:77–117.
144. Muller SC, Hsieh JT, Lue TF, Tanagho EA. Castration and erection. An animal study. Eur Urol 1988; 15:118–24.
145. Kimura K, Hashine K, Tamura M et al. Effect of testosterone on contraction and relaxation of isolated human corpus cavernosum tissue. Int J Impot Res 1990; 2(Suppl 1):53.
146. Andersson KE, Holmquist F, Bodker A. Castration enhances NANC nerve-mediated relaxation in rabbit isolated corpus cavernosum. Acta Physiol Scand 1992; 3:155–72.
147. Holmquist F, Persson K, Bodker A, Andersson KE. Some pre- and postjunctional effects of castration in rabbit isolated corpus cavernosum and urethra. J Urol 1994; 152:1011–16.
148. Giuliano F, Rampin O, Schirar A et al. Autonomic control of penile erection: modulation by testosterone in the rat. J Neuroendocrinol 1993; 5:677–83.
149. Carani C, Granata ARM, Faustini Fustini M, Marrama P. Prolactin and testosterone: their role in male sexual function. Int J Androl 1996; 19:48–54.
150. Carroll JL, Ellis D, Bagley DH. Impotence in the elderly. Evaluation of erectile failure in men older than seventy years of age. Jefferson Sexual Function Center. Urology 1992; 39:226–30.
151. Feldman HA, Goldstein I, Hatzichristou DG et al. Impotence and its medical and psychosocial correlates: results of the Massachusetts Male Aging Study. J Urol 1994; 151:54–61.
152. McCulloch DK, Campbell IW, Wu FC et al. The prevalence of diabetic impotence. Diabetologia 1980; 18:279–83.
153. Jensen SB. Diabetic sexual dysfunction; a comparative study of 160 insulin treated diabetic men and women and an age-matched control group. Arch Sex Behav 1981; 10(6):493–504.

154. Michal V. Arterial disease as a cause of impotence. Clin Endocrinol Metab 1982; 11:725–48.

155. Lincoln J, Crowe R, Blacklay PE et al. Changes in the vipergic, cholinergic, and adrenergic innervation of human penile tissue in diabetics and non diabetic impotent males. J Urol 1987; 137:1053.

156. Blanco R, de Tejada SI, Goldstein I et al. Dysfunctional penile cholinergic nerves in diabetic impotent men. J Urol 1992; 144:278–80.

157. Bemelmans BL, Meuleman EJ, Doesburg WH et al. Erectile dysfunction in diabetic men: the neurological factor revisited. J Urol 1994; 151:884–9.

158. Benvenuti F, Boncinelli L, Vignoli GC. Male sexual impotence in diabetes mellitus: vasculogenic versus neurogenic factors. Neurourol Urodynam 1993; 12:145–51; discussion, 152.

159. Yamaguchi Y, Kumamoto Y. [Etiological analysis of male diabetic erectile dysfunction with particular emphasis on findings of vascular and neurological examinations]. [in Japanese]. Nippon Hinyokika Gakkai Zasshi – Japanese Journal of Urology 1994; 85:1474–83.

160. Veves A, Webster L, Chen TF et al. Aetiopathogenesis and management of impotence in diabetic males: four years experience from a combined clinic. Diabet Med 1995; 12:77–82.

161. Azadzoi KM, Saenz deTejada I. Diabetes mellitus impairs neurogenic and endothelium-dependent relaxation of rabbit corpus cavernosum smooth muscle. J Urol 1992; 148:1587–91.

162. Jeremy JY, Thompson CS, Mikhailidis DP, Dandona P. Experimental diabetes mellitus inhibits prostacyclin synthesis by the rat penis: pathological implications. Diabetologia 1985; 28:365–8.

163. Dyck PJ, Lambert EH, Windebank AJ. Acute hyperosmolar hyperglycaemia causes axonal shrinkage and reduced nerve conduction velocity. Exp Neurol 1981; 71:507.

164. Virag R, Bouilly P, Frydman D. Is impotence an arterial disorder? A study of arterial risk factors in 440 impotent men. Lancet 1985; i:181–4.

165. Shabsigh R, Fishman IJ, Schum C, Dunn JK. Cigarette smoking and other vascular risk factors in vasculogenic impotence. Urology 1991; 38:227–31.

166. Sullivan ME, Thompson CS, Dashwood MR, Khan MA, Jeremy JY, Morgan RJ et al. Nitric oxide and penile erection: is erectile dysfunction another manifestation of vascular diseae? Cardiovasc Res 1999; 43(3):658–665.

167. Vane JR, Anggard EE, Botting RM. Regulatory functions of the vascular endothelium. N Engl J Med 1990; 323(1):27–36.

168. Pegge N, Twomey M, Ramsey M, Vaughton K, Price D. Autonomic and Endothelial Function are Impaired in Erectile Dysfunction but do Not Predict Response to Sildenafil. Diabet Med 2001; 18(Suppl 2):89.

169. Bulpitt CJ, Dollery CT, Carne S. Changes in symptoms of hypertensive patients after referral to hospital clinic. Br Heart J 1976; 38:121.

170. Virag R. Impotence: a new field in angiography. Internat Angiol 1984; 3:217–19.

171. Ralph DR, Pryor JP. Veno-occlusive dysfunction: a cavernosal smooth muscle pathology? Curr Opin Urol 1996; 6:83–6.
172. Campbell WB, Johnson AR, Callahan KS, Graham RM. Anti-platelet activity of beta-adrenergic antagonists: inhibition of thromboxane synthesis and platelet aggregation in patients receiving long-term propranolol treatment. Lancet 1981; 11:1382–4.
173. Mikhailidis DP, Barradas MA, Mier A et al. Platelet function in patients admitted with a diagnosis of myocardial infarction. Angiology 1987; 38:36–45.
174. Hogan MJ, Wallin JD, Baer RM. Antihypertensive therapy and male sexual dysfunction. Psychosomatics 1980; 21:234.
175. Kochar MS, Zeller JR, Itskovitz H. Prazosin in hypertension with and without methyldopa. Clin Pharm Ther 1979; 25:143.
176. Pitts NE. A clinical evaluation of prazosin, a new antihypertensive agent. Postgrad Med 1975; 58:117.
177. Abrams HS, Hester LR, Sheridan WF, Epstein GM. Sexual functioning in patients with chronic renal failure. J Nerv Ment Dis 1975; 160:220–6.
178. Gittes RF, Waters WB. Sexual impotence and overlooked complications of a second renal transplant. J Urol 1979; 121:718.
179. Jeremy JY, Mikhailidis DP, Thompson CS, Dandona P. The effect of cigarette smoke and diabetes mellitus on muscarinic stimulation of prostacyclin synthesis by the rat penis. Diabetes Res 1986; 3:467–9.
180. Hirshkowitz M, Karacan I, Howell JW et al. Nocturnal penile tumescence in cigarette smokers with erectile dysfunction. Urology 1992; 39:101–7.
181. Wei M, Macera CA, Davis DR et al. Total cholesterol and high density lipoprotein cholesterol as important predictors of erectile dysfunction. Am J Epidemiol 1994; 140:930–7.
182. Christ GJ, Spray DC, Brink PR. Characterization of K currents in cultured human corporal smooth muscle cells. J Androl 1993; 14(5):319–28.
183. Giuliano FA, Rampin O, Benoit G, Jardin A. Neural control of penile erection. Urol Clin North Am 1995; 22(4):747–66.
184. Christ GJ. The penis as a vascular organ. The importance of corporal smooth muscle tone in the control of erection. Urol Clin North Am 1995; 22(4):727–45.

chapter 3

Epidemiology and clinical features of erectile dysfunction in diabetes

William D Alexander

Introduction

Impotence has long been recognised as being associated with diabetes. John Rollo recorded in 1798 – '... A 30 year old Glaswegian porter, father of several children but since he has been seized with diabetes – "Coitus nullus. Erigitum nunquam: ne quidem semel rigescit".'[1] Whether your Latin is adequate for full translation or not, this eloquent phrase must surely not only conjure up sympathy but a determination to try and do something to help such a distressing incapacity. Sadly it was to be almost 200 years before diabetes care teams included the management of erectile dysfunction amongst their routine services.

Prevalence of erectile dysfunction

The prevalence of impotence in the general male population is estimated to be approximately 10%. This prevalence increases with age. The Kinsey report in 1948 reported the prevalence of erectile dysfunction as 5% in 40-year-old men, 10% in 60-year-old men and 20% in 70-year-old men.[2]

In more recent times the Massachusetts Male Aging Study suggested a similar rate, for complete erectile failure, of 9.6% in men aged 40–70, 5% in men aged 40 years and 15% in those aged 70 years.[3] A survey by The Impotence Association in the United Kingdom (1998) estimated that 2–3 million British men suffer from impotence and that only a minority receive any form of treatment.[4]

Recognition of the frequency of significant erectile dysfunction amongst *diabetic men* is now generally agreed to be considerably higher, and it probably affects around 35% of all diabetic men over the age of 18 years. In reviews of the subject, Eardley and Gale[5] quoted rates between 23 and 59% and Bancroft and Gutierrez 35–55% in the hospital setting.[6] Hackett, in a survey of 428 diabetic men from 10 general practices, found a prevalence rate of 55%, of whom 39% suffered from the problem all of the time.[7] This was significantly higher than in a non-diabetic control group, of whom 26% had some problems with erections and 5% suffered the problem all of the time.

The prevalence of impotence in diabetic men increases significantly with age. McCulloch et al.[8] found a prevalence of 5.7% in men aged 20–24 years, which rose to 52.4% in men aged 55–59 years. Similar figures were found by Cummings and Alexander[9] and Price et al.[10] (Fig. 3.1). The reason why erectile dysfunction increases more with advancing years is not known, but is probably related to the increasing likelihood of other complications of the diabetes and other significant aggravating conditions, particularly vascular disease and the need for antihypertensive drugs. One large study has suggested the prevalence of erectile dysfunction is greater in type II than type I diabetes (51% vs. 37%).[11]

In most diabetes care services, the majority of people will have type II diabetes and the average age of men attending will be over 50 years of age. It is likely therefore that a large proportion of the men attending any diabetes care service will suffer with erectile

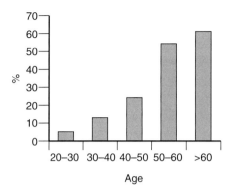

Figure 3.1 *Prevalence of erectile dysfunction by age of a diabetic clinic population.*[10]

dysfunction, and therefore it should be essential that involved health care professionals should have an understanding of the problem and its management.

Is erectile dysfunction a diabetic complication?

Whether erectile dysfunction is directly related to diabetes itself and its specific complications, or is more related to associated factors and conditions, has been controversial in the past and is explored in depth in Chapter 2.

Studies of men attending clinics for other medical disorders suggest that the prevalence of erectile dysfunction specifically due to diabetes per se may be less frequent than that due to other causes related to the many associated conditions that affect men with type II diabetes (noninsulin-dependent diabetes mellitus or NIDDM). This particularly applies to men with multiple vascular risk factors or overt vascular disease in whom both the condition and some of the treatments will have a significant effect on erectile function. One study of men attending a medical outpatient clinic revealed, by questionnaire, that whereas 23% of those with diabetes suffered erectile dysfunction, 20% of non-diabetic attenders also had a problem. In the oldest age group (40–60 years), the relative prevalence was 28% in the diabetic group and 30% in the others.[12] Slag et al. also reported a high prevalence of erectile dysfunction of 34% amongst 1180 men attending a general medical clinic.[13]

This all suggests that the prevalence of erectile dysfunction in type II diabetes may be much higher because the men are in an older age group and often suffer from other conditions (and treatments) that predispose them, both psychologically and physically, to the problem. This does not of course alter the fact that men attending diabetes services have a high prevalence of erectile dysfunction and that such services should be able to provide advice and management. It does, however, cast doubt as to whether diabetes per se, particularly type II, is such a common cause, and the term 'diabetic impotence' should be avoided.

In type I diabetes erectile dysfunction is more likely to be specifically related to the diabetes and to its duration and degree of metabolic control as well as to microvascular complications.

Ascertainment in diabetic men

The prevalence of erectile dysfunction may also be seriously underestimated if men are relied upon to volunteer the problem, as many men remain embarrassed or ashamed to do so. Alexander and Evans found a volunteered prevalence of 7% amongst men (under 60 years of age) attending a hypertension clinic who were asked whether they were suffering any side effects from the antihypertensive drug methyldopa.[14] However, a much higher prevalence of 50% was found when the same men answered a questionnaire that specifically addressed the question of impotence. Price has justifiably described erectile dysfunction as 'the most neglected complication of diabetes' because, despite this high prevalence, its management has been largely ignored by diabetes care services until recent years.[15]

Undoubtedly, many men suffer in silence and do not present at all. Studies in medical clinics that have used questionnaires to ascertain the prevalence of the condition have received far higher rates than those acquired by people volunteering the problem.[14] This may be because of embarrassment or lack of knowledge about the subject, which until recently has been seldom discussed either between men themselves or within the media. Although publicity has increased enormously, it will still often only be detected by health care professionals with an interest in erectile dysfunction.

A survey on behalf of the Impotence Association[4] showed that only a minority of all men with erectile dysfunction received any form of treatment; 86% of men had sought advice from lay sources instead of visiting their general practitioner, and 41% had spent a significant amount of money in their quest for information and treatment before or instead of using the National Health Service. Of those who sought help in primary care, 49% considered the help they received inadequate.

Hackett in his study of primary care found that 40% of diabetic men and 50% of controls had not discussed the problem with anyone.[7] Despite regular attendances at their diabetic clinics, only 33% of sufferers had discussed the problem with a general practitioner.

It has been said that men may be embarrassed to discuss the problem with a health care professional and also that they may be more likely to mention it to a female specialist nurse than a man. A study by Cummings et al. tends to refute this, in that only 17% said they would be embarrassed to discuss the problem, but this was more likely to be so if they were seeing a female member of staff rather than a man (37% vs. 12%).[16] Like many other studies, this one also showed poor satisfaction rates, with 33% not being offered any treatment at all and 55% finding the management of the problem unsatisfactory.

Quality of life issues

Erectile dysfunction can significantly affect quality of life. The Impotence Association survey found psychological symptoms of lowered self-esteem and depression in 62% of men; 40% expressed concern with either new or established relationships and 21% blamed it for the break-up of a relationship.[4] The survey reported that many doctors appeared reluctant to be proactive, even when patients presented themselves to primary care for help. Further analysis of this problem in Hackett's series[7] showed that 45% of diabetic men stated that they thought about their erectile dysfunction all or most of the time compared with 23% of non-diabetic men; 23% felt that it severely affected their quality of life and 10% that it severely affected their relationship with their partner. A further finding in this study suggested that 80% would like to seek advice and treatment from their doctor if an effective and acceptable treatment was available. There appeared to be a consistent finding that diabetic men and their partners were more affected by the loss of erectile function that non-diabetic controls.

Cummings et al. showed that 38% of diabetic men with erectile dysfunction felt their relationship had suffered moderately and 19% severely; 91% would like to seek medical advice if effective treatment was available.[16] However, 46% of these men were unaware that treatment was available and in only 17% had a health care professional spontaneously discussed the problem. Of those who were aware, the information they had obtained had largely been from sources other than primary care or hospital health care professionals; it was mainly from newspapers, magazines, television and the British Diabetic Association (now Diabetes UK) magazine. In this particular group of patients, those who had discussed the problem were more likely to have done so with their general practitioner (65%) than with the hospital clinic (35%). It was interesting that, although 92% of these men said they would consider asking their partners to attend an advice and treatment clinic with them, the experience of most people running clinics is that fewer than 25% actually do bring their partners. Whether this is because men don't actually ask, or their partners refuse, is unknown.

These findings show that there is still a long way to go to improve the service to diabetic men and their partners who are suffering with erectile dysfunction.

To screen or not to screen
The above findings also raise the question as to whether there should be routine screening for erectile dysfunction within the diabetes clinic, perhaps as a part of the annual diabetes review. Different centres

have different philosophies, but it is important that if there is to be an active screening programme then this should be backed up by an active assessment and treatment programme within, or agreed and available to, the department that screens. Screening will identify a large number of sufferers but not necessarily a large number of people who require treatments.

Alexander[18] found that whereas 88% of men who had volunteered a problem of erectile dysfunction proceeded to active treatment, only 18% did so who had been identified as a result of answering positively to a questionnaire. It may be of course that such numbers would be considerably higher if treatments became more acceptable. An alternative to active screening, and perhaps a more time- and cost-effective method, is to have a good awareness programme in diabetes units using posters and educational leaflets. Men, and indeed their partners, will thereby be made aware that the service is not only aware of the existence of the problem but also that it has the where-withal to offer treatment. Educational leaflets will enable men to find out what treatments involve and, where appropriate, discuss this further with their partners.

Clinical presentation and assessment

The majority of diabetic men will present with true erectile dysfunction of varying degrees. Others, however, may have other problems related both to the penis itself or sexual function generally and these need to be considered. Such problems may be physical and/or psychological and include:

- congenital abnormalities
- curvature, e.g. Peyronie's disease
- balanitis and phimosis
- ejaculatory abnormalities – premature, delayed or retrograde
- misconceptions of 'normality'
- psychosexual problems
- lack of libido.

Men will vary in their perception of what the word impotence means, and if a direct questioning approach is adopted it is important that the question is clear:

- 'Do you suffer from impotence?' is rather threatening and demeaning.
- 'Do you suffer from any sexual difficulties?' is probably too broad and could raise many problems that are completely out of the problem-solving abilities of the questioner.
- 'Do you have any problem with your erections' should be sufficiently explicit and could be preceded by a softer approach such as 'Do you have any other problems you would like to discuss?'.

If it is clear that there is a problem then more in depth questions and discussion should ensue. This is particularly important if such men are then referred on to a different specialist because, unless the exact problem is identified, a totally inappropriate referral may be made.

Clinical history

The history of the presentation of the problem of erectile dysfunction is the most important part of the assessment process. It is important not only to establish exactly what the problem is but also to find the likely causes in order to be able to give a reasoned explanation of the problem to the patient. In a significant number of men this is all that is required, as they will not wish to pursue treatment options.

Erectile dysfunction in diabetic men is usually gradual in onset and progressive in nature. Often the earliest feature is the inability to sustain an erection long enough for satisfactory intercourse. This may be intermittent initially. Loss of erectile function of sudden onset is often stated to indicate a psychogenic cause but there is little evidence to support this. Similarly, preservation of spontaneous and early morning erections does not necessarily indicate a psychogenic cause.

Loss of libido is consistent with hypogonadism but is not a reliable symptom. In many societies the expression of a high sex drive is not encouraged, whereas celibacy and asceticism are lauded. Thus, many men will understate their sex drive for a variety of reasons, including guilt. Others suppress their libidos as a defence mechanism to prevent the disappointment of failure. A history obtained from the partner without the patient present often reveals interesting and useful insight into the problem.

A full medical history should also be obtained, as this may reveal potential causes of sexual dysfunction, such as cardiovascular disease and hypertension. For the same reason a full drug history is essential.

Standard questions that may be asked of men might include:

- *What exactly is the problem?*
Failure to obtain and/or sustain an erection. Presence or absence of spontaneous or self-stimulated erections. Is it a different problem such as ejaculatory disorder, Peyronie's disease, lack of libido? How long has it been a problem, how did it start and how has it progressed?

- *What do you think is the likely cause?*
It is worth asking men for their views on cause. In some men there may be a definite relationship to the onset of certain conditions or the initiation of medication(s). It is also worth asking: 'Do you think it is mainly physical or psychological?' In considering psychological aspects, it is helpful to discuss predisposing, precipitating, potentiating and perpetuating factors.

- *Why is it a problem and what is your partner's attitude?*
Assessment should include a discussion of sexual function in general and relationship issues in particular. It is most helpful to invite the partner, if possible, to attend with the man, although most men prefer to attend alone initially.

- *What do you know about possible treatments and how would you like to proceed?*
Some men will be aware of various treatments, whereas others may have no idea at all. It is important to discuss all options, using demonstration models if possible.

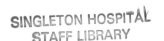

It has been traditional to consider psychological versus physical causes. Although this will not always affect the final choice of treatment, it may be useful in explaining the nature of the condition and the most appropriate management pathways. It is unlikely that men with pure organic erectile dysfunction will benefit at all from a psychological approach, and it would be inappropriate and unacceptably intrusive to refer many such men down such a route. It may also be inappropriate only to initiate treatment to restore erection of the penis when psychological problems predominate, thereby ignoring psychological aspects and a man's relationship with his partner and their relevance and significance. That is not to say that men with predominantly psychological causes will not benefit from physical treatments or vice versa.

Table 3.1 lists the factors that traditionally have been quoted to help to distinguish physical from psychological erectile dysfunction.

The classic presentation of an organic problem might be a man in his 60s with type II diabetes, who has smoked for years, has perhaps had a significant cardiovascular event and is on antihypertensive medication. He has noticed over the past few years an initial reduction in rigidity of erection followed by a gradual onset of increasing

Table 3.1 Factors that help distinguish physical from psychological erectile dysfunction

Physical factors	Psychological factors
Gradual onset	Sudden onset
Persistent and consistent	Intermittent and 'partner variable'
No spontaneous or self-stimulated response	Spontaneous/self-stimulated erections occur
No overt psychological problems	Overt psychological problems
Significant physical problems	No significant physical factors

inability to sustain it and latterly a complete absence of any erectile function at all. Such a problem may be further compounded by his partner suffering some health problems and perhaps a gynaecological intervention or two that has prevented any sexual activity for a year or so. Restoration of the requirement for penetrative intercourse may occur with the recovery of the partner and perhaps the introduction of hormone replacement therapy or alternatively a new relationship with a sexually active partner.

It is often said that restoration of erections for penetrative intercourse is not necessary for sexual fulfilment and that sexual counselling regarding other methods of satisfaction might be employed. This might be acceptable to a few but is often considered totally unacceptable behaviour by many men (and their partners) of the older generations.

Physical examination

As part of the physical examination the patient's overall physical condition should be assessed not only to give insight into the aetiology of erectile dysfunction but also into the choice of treatment. Poor manual dexterity or a large protuberant abdomen may preclude the use of vacuum devices or self-injection therapy. It is also important to elicit any symptoms or signs of depression, as this is a potentially treatable cause of erectile dysfunction.

The condition of the external genitalia should be assessed carefully for the presence of a phimosis or Peyronie's disease. Examination should include an estimation of testicular volume and assessment of other features to suggest hypogonadism. The need for a full general examination will depend on clues elicited during the history.

Who should provide a management service?

A recent survey of diabetologists in the UK reported that 36% routinely asked men if they had any erection problems and although 98% considered that treatment for erectile dysfunction should be provided within a diabetes service, 50% did not actually offer any treatment themselves but referred men on to other specialists, mainly urologists (O'Malley and Price, pers comm, 1996). It does seem odd that practitioners in a specialty that publicises its asset of a multidisciplinary and holistic approach, and who get to know their patients so well over the years, refer them to a surgical stranger for a medical treatment when they have finally summoned up the courage to mention one of their most intimate problems!

Ideally, there should be a multidisciplinary team working together that includes physicians, andrologists, nurses, psychologists and sex therapists. Although this is the case in a few larger centres, it is not possible in most units: if not practicable, there should at least be local availability and agreed referral pathways between such people, even if it is not possible to be working together under the same roof.

Summary

Erectile dysfunction is a common problem in diabetic men and has a significant effect on quality of life. Its cause is usually multifactorial. There is currently a significant degree of dissatisfaction about available management services. The multidisciplinary nature of diabetes care services, and the increasing recognition of the importance of the problem should stimulate diabetes teams to provide an assessment and treatment service themselves. Awareness programmes are recommended to encourage those men, or their partners, who have a problem and wish to receive help, to mention their problem. The essential part of the clinical assessment is the history and relatively simple-structured questioning that will ascertain what the problem is, what its likely cause may be and what is the most appropriate course of action.

References

1.   Rollo J. An account of two cases of diabetes mellitus: with remarks as they arose during the process of care. John Rollo's book. London: C Dilly, 1798.
2.   Kinsey AC, Pomeroy WB, Martin CE. Sexual behaviour in the human male. Philadelphia: W.B. Saunders, 1948.
3.   Feldman HA, Johannes CB, Derby CA et al. Erectile dysfunction and coronary risk factors: prospective results from the Massachusetts male aging study. Preventive Medicine 2000; 30(4):328–38.
4.   Craig A. One in Ten. London: Impotence Association, 1998.
5.   Eardley I, Gale E. Diabetic impotence. In: Kirby RS, Carson CC, Webster GD, eds. Impotence Diagnosis and Management of Erectile Dysfunction. Butterworth-Heinemann, 2001.
6.   Bancroft J, Gutierrez P. Erectile dysfunction in men with and without diabetes mellitus: a comparative study. Diabet Med 1996; 13(1):84–9.
7.   Hackett G. Impotence – the most neglected complication of diabetes. Diabet Res 1995.
8.   McCulloch DK, Campbell IW, Wu FC, Prescott RJ, Clarke BF. The prevalence of diabetic impotence. Diabetologia 1980; 18(4):279–83.
9.   Cummings MH, Alexander WD. Erectile dysfunction in patients with diabetes. Hosp Med 1999; 60(9):638–44.
10. Price D, O'Malley BP, James MA, Roshan M, Hearnshaw JR. Why are impotent diabetic men not being treated. Pract Diabet 1991; 8:10–11.
11. Fedele D, Coscelli C, Santeusanio F et al. Erectile dysfunction in diabetic subjects in Italy. Gruppo Italiano Studio Deficit Erettile nei Diabetici. Diabet Care 1998; 21(11):1973–7.
12. Lester E, Grant AJ, Woodroffe FJ. Impotence in diabetic and non-diabetic hospital outpatients. Br Med J 1980; 281(6236):354–5.
13. Slag MF, Morley JE, Elson MK et al. Impotence in medical clinic outpatients. JAMA 1983; 249(13):1736–40.
14. Alexander WD, Evans JI. Letter: side effects of methyldopa. Br Med J 1975; 2(5969):501.
15. Price DE. Managing impotence in diabetes. Br Med J 1993; 307(6899):275–6.
16. Cummings MH, Meeking D, Warburton F, Alexander WD. The diabetic male's perception of erectile dysfunction. Pract Diabet Internat 1997; 14(4):100–2.
17. Dunsmuir WD, Holmes SA. The aetiology and management of erectile, ejaculatory, and fertility problems in men with diabetes mellitus. Diabet Med 1996; 13(8):700–8.
18. Alexander WD. The diabetes physician and an assessment and treatment programme for male erectile impotence. Diabet Med 1990; 7(6):540–3.

chapter 4

Management of impotence in diabetes

David E Price, Mitra Boollel and Nandan Koppiker

Assessment and investigation of erectile dysfunction in diabetes

Investigation of erectile dysfunction

Many factors contribute to the development of erectile dysfunction in diabetes, so a physician treating an impotent diabetic man has the choice of a wide range of potential investigations. These include tests of vascular, neuronal and hormonal function as well as tests of spontaneous erectile activity. While the investigation of erectile dysfunction may be important, it is no substitute for a good history and examination, as described in Chapter 3. In most cases after a good clinical assessment, few investigations are required.

Investigation of spontaneous and nocturnal erections

Until the 1980s it was received wisdom to determine whether erectile dysfunction was 'psychogenic' or 'physical' in origin; consequently, a variety of techniques were developed to determine if nocturnal and early morning erections were maintained on the basis this would indicate a psychogenic cause. Equipment was developed to measure tumescence at home during sleep and also in the laboratory under conditions of sexual stimulation. One of the more sophisticated such devices is the 'RigiScan' (Dacomed Corporation, Minneapolis, USA), a computerised device which measures the circumference and rigidity of the penis.[1] At the other end of the scale, a ring of postage stamps applied around the penis was used as a cheap alternative. If the ring was broken in the morning it was assumed tumescence had occurred during the night.

It is now widely accepted that to divide impotence into categories such as physical or psychogenic is unhelpful, particularly in diabetes. Impotence has a physical component in the vast majority of diabetic men, and erectile function rarely improves without a physical treatment.[2,3] In addition, there may be a superimposed or secondary psychological problem such as performance anxiety. Thus, almost all diabetic men with erectile dysfunction require both a physical and psychological approach to treatment. Nocturnal penile tumescence and rigidity studies are useful research tools but are not helpful in the routine management of erectile dysfunction.

Assessment of vascular function

Both arterial insufficiency and venous dysfunction can contribute to the development of erectile dysfunction in diabetes. Various investigations have been developed to assess both arterial inflow and veno-occlusive mechanisms. These include cavernosometry, radionuclear scintigraphy and cavernous oxygen tension.[4] Most of these investigations are cumbersome, time-consuming and not readily available. Furthermore, arterial reconstruction is rarely of benefit in the management of erectile dysfunction in diabetic men (see below). 'Venous leak' surgery is controversial but is probably of limited benefit. Therefore, the investigation of vascular dysfunction rarely alters management and has little role to play in the management of diabetic men with erectile dysfunction.

Neuronal function

Autonomic dysfunction plays a central role in the development of erectile dysfunction in diabetes. Unfortunately, no simple reliable test of pelvic autonomic function exists. Many autonomic function tests have been described; most are measures of cardiac autonomic dysfunction, such as the heart rate response to deep breathing or the Valsalva manoevre. These are well-established tests but they do not necessarily reflect pelvic autonomic dysfunction. There have been several attempts to develop tests of pelvic autonomic and somatic neuropathy, including sacral evoked-potential testing,[5,6] bulbocavernosus electromyography and dorsal nerve somatosensory-evoked potential testing.[6] These tests, although time-consuming and cumbersome, are useful as research tools, but it is unlikely they have a role in the routine management of erectile dysfunction in diabetic men.

Intracorporeal injection as a test

An intracavernosal test dose of a vasoactive drug has been advocated as a useful test of penile vascularity. The logic is appealing; if a satisfactory erection can be obtained following the injection of a pharmacological agent then there cannot be too much wrong with the blood supply to the erectile tissue and injection therapy might be an appropriate treatment. This may well be true, but no conclusions can be drawn from failure to respond as many men with normal nocturnal tumescence studies fail to get an erection after an intracorporeal papaverine injection.[7] This may be due to the inhibitory effects of being nervous and anxious in a totally artificial testing situation.

There is no evidence that performing an intracorporeal test injection is of any value in the investigation of an impotent diabetic man. If a man is considering self-injection therapy as a treatment option, it is certainly worth considering giving him a test intracorporeal injection so that he knows what the process will involve. However, as an investigation, it rarely gives any useful information about the aetiology of the erectile dysfunction and does not predict whether a patient will respond to self-treatment at home.

Endocrine function

Gonadal function has a central role in the development and maintenance of sexual function in man, and hypogonadism is an uncommon but important cause of erectile dysfunction as it is usually treatable (Tables 4.1). It also leads to loss of libido and it is often the partner of a man with hypogonadism who persuades him to seek help. The relationship between androgen levels and male libido and sexual function is complex and poorly understood. In general, hypo-gonadism is associated with reduced libido and erectile dysfunction. However, some men with castrate serum levels of testosterone have normal libidos and adequate erectile function.[8,9] Clearly, diabetic men are not immune from developing hypogonadism but is there any relationship between diabetes and gonadal function? In rats diabetes causes a reduction in serum testosterone levels[10] but subnormal serum testosterone levels have not consistently been reported in impotent diabetic men. The available evidence suggests there is probably not a significant relationship between diabetes and hypogonadism. Thus, we should only assess gonadal function in diabetic men with erectile dysfunction if it is considered worthwhile to look for a coincidental problem causing hypogonadism.

Common sense dictates that serum testosterone and probably prolactin estimation should be done if the clinical picture suggests a

Table 4.1 Endocrine causes of erectile dysfunction

- Primary hypogonadism
    orchitis
    Klinefelter's syndrome
    castration
    renal failure
- Secondary hypogonadism
    pituitary tumour
    prolactinoma
    haemochromatosis
- Acromegaly
- Thyroid disease

pituitary tumour or any other possible cause of hypogonadism. It is controversial, however, if a hormonal screen should be undertaken in all diabetic men with erectile dysfunction. Buvat and Lemaire reported that the serum testosterone was subnormal in 107 out of 1022 men with erectile dysfunction but 40% were normal on repeat.[9] Two pituitary tumours and one prolactinoma were discovered after testosterone determination. In most cases the subnormal testosterone was due to what the authors described as 'hypothalamic dysfunction'. Androgen therapy produced improvement in erectile function in 16 out of 44 (36%) men with subnormal serum testosterone. They concluded that in the investigation of erectile dysfunction, serum testosterone should be measured routinely in all men over 50 years and in those under 50 with reduced libido or abnormal physical examination. The authors also suggested serum prolactin should only be measured if the serum testosterone is low or if reduced libido or gynaecomastia are present.

There are few similar data for diabetic men with erectile dysfunction but it would seem likely that the prevalence of hypogonadism is little different.

Summary

The majority of diabetic men will develop erectile dysfunction, and in most cases it will be due to the diabetes or a related pathology. Knowing the exact pathogenesis rarely alters management. Any physician treating

---

Table 4.2 Investigation of erectile dysfunction in diabetes

- Assessment of cardiovascular risk and disease status
- Serum testosterone if libido reduced
- Serum prolactin and lutenising hormone (LH) if testosterone is subnormal
- Glycosylated haemoglobin, electrolytes, blood count, liver function tests if clinically indicated

impotence should exclude a treatable cause of impotence and address concomitant problems such as poor metabolic control and cardiovascular status. The investigations that should be considered in the management of erectile dysfunction in diabetes are listed in Table 4.2.

General advice for the impotent man and his partner

Most diabetic men and their partners seeking treatment for impotence are middle aged and have been married for many years, often longer than their physician, and, like all patients, should be treated with respect and dignity.[11] In most cases they have had a good sex life prior to the development of erectile dysfunction and do not need advice about the role of sex in their relationship. It is particularly unhelpful to tell them that it is possible to have a fulfilling relationship without penetrative sex. It is up to them to decide how important penetrative sex is and they must not be made to feel guilty for wanting it.

It is particularly important to establish whether the patient and his partner have a good relationship. Some couples will seek a treatment for erectile dysfunction in an attempt to save a failing relationship. Anecdotal experience has suggested that restoring a man's potency in this situation is rarely successful and is more likely to make things worse as it introduces a new tension into the relationship. The assistance of a suitably qualified psychosexual counsellor should be considered in this situation.

If a couple is to be offered a physical treatment for impotence it is important to establish that they have a positive attitude to it. They should be encouraged to use the treatment together. Occasionally a man will want to conceal the use of the impotence treatment from his partner; this rarely succeeds and should be discouraged.

General health advice
Erectile dysfunction is an independent risk factor for cardiovascular disease and can be the presenting symptom of diabetes. The initial

Table 4.3 Medications and drugs associated with sexual dysfunction

Antihypertensives
- Thiazide diuretics
- Beta blockers
- Calcium channel blockers
- ACE inhibitors
- Central sympatholytics (methyldopa, clonidine)

Antidepressants
- Tricyclics
- Monoamine oxidase inhibitors

Note: Selective serotonin re-uptake inhibitors (SSRIs) can cause ejaculatory problems

Major tranquillisers
- Phenothiazines
- Haloperidol

Hormones
- Luteinising hormone releasing hormone (goserilin, buserilin)
- Oestrogens (stilboestrol)
- Anti-androgens (cyproterone)

Miscellaneous
- 5-alpha reductase inhibitors (finasteride)
- Statins (simvastatin, atorvastatin, pravastatin)
- Cimetidine
- Digoxin
- Metoclopramide

Drugs of abuse
- Alcohol
- Tobacco
- Marijuana
- Amphetamines
- Anabolic steroids
- Barbiturates
- Opiates

consultation for erectile dysfunction provides an opportunity for screening and to address other medical problems. If diabetic control is poor the patient should be given advice to improve it; however, poor control should not be used as a reason not to offer treatment. There is an association between smoking and erectile dysfunction and all patients who smoke should be advised to stop for reasons of general health, although there is no evidence that stopping will improve erectile function. Similarly, there is no evidence that reducing alcohol intake will improve erectile function.

Many diabetic men will be taking drugs for other medical conditions and many of these are associated with erectile dysfunction (Table 4.3). In particular, antihypertensive agents are commonly used in diabetes and are particularly associated with impotence. Of these, thiazide diuretics and beta blockers are the commonest offenders, whereas alpha blockers are the least likely to cause impotence. There is always a strong temptation to try and change treatment to improve sexual function. However, experience has shown it is usually a fruitless activity in diabetic men and is not advisable unless there is a strong temporal relationship between starting treatment and the onset of erectile dysfunction.

Counselling

Introduction

It is hard to overestimate the influence of the work of Masters and Johnson on the development of counselling in the treatment of sexual dysfunction. They were amongst the first to systematically study sexual function and dysfunction in human subjects for which they deserve great credit. In their original seminal work, they reported that of 213 men, only seven had a physiological cause for their erectile dysfunction.[12] From this the belief entered medical folklore that impotence had a psychogenic cause in 95% of cases. Even though Masters and Johnson studied a selected population very different to that seen by most diabetologists, psychosexual counselling was advocated as the most important treatment for erectile dysfunction in diabetes. It wasn't until the new development of effective physical treatments, such as self-injection therapy, that it was widely accepted that counselling alone was not sufficient in most diabetic men with erectile dysfunction.

The role of psychosexual counselling in the impotent diabetic man

The distinction must be drawn between specialist counselling given by a psychosexual counsellor and the explanation and advice that all physicians should give their patients. Few would dispute the latter form of counselling is essential, but the importance of specialist counselling in the management of erectile dysfunction in diabetes is more controversial. Prior to the development of effective physical treatments, many diabetic men and their partners underwent many sessions over several weeks of psychosexual counselling involving techniques such as sensate focusing. This was time-consuming, expensive and, more importantly, gave the couple the impression that the answer to their problem was in their own hands, which often created feelings of guilt if the treatment was unsuccessful.

Few controlled studies have been done to examine whether psychosexual counselling is of benefit in erectile dysfunction. In one of the few studies in diabetic men, McCulloch et al. reported that psychosexual counselling produced long-term benefit in only 3 out of 20 diabetic men, none of whom were identified from pre-treatment characteristics.[3] Spontaneous recovery of erectile function is very unusual in diabetic men, and most will require a physical treatment if they wish to achieve penetrative sexual function.[2] There is no evidence that simply treating the patient with one of the physical treatments without formal counselling does any harm, even if there is a large psychogenic component to the problem. Several published series have suggested that diabetologists can offer treatment for erectile dysfunction with good results without the assistance of counsellors.[11,13–16] Whether a better service could be offered to diabetic patients with the assistance of specialist counsellors is not known, but in the past many physicians have been deterred from offering treatment for erectile dysfunction to their diabetic patients because they have not had access to counselling services.

Referral to a psychosexual counsellor should be considered if there is any suggestion of problems in the relationship, depression, severe anxiety, loss of attraction between partners, fear of intimacy or marked performance anxiety. These problems are not particularly common in diabetic men, as generally they are middle-aged and have long-standing relationships. However, any physician who treats diabetic men with erectile dysfunction will from time to time have to deal with couples with some of these problems and should not be deterred from taking them on. Common sense is usually all that is needed to decide if further counselling is necessary, and the couple will often know themselves if it would be useful. If in doubt, little harm can be done by offering one of the physical treatments for impotence, provided there is no tension in the relationship.

Summary

Most diabetic men and their partners seeking help for erectile dysfunction are middle-aged and have been in a stable relationship for many years. In most cases psychosexual counselling is not required; it is important to establish that the couple has maintained a good relationship and to give common-sense advice.

Vacuum therapy

History

In 1917 the United States Patent Office issued a patent to Otto Lederer for a device that allowed 'persons considered to be completely impotent to perform sexual intercourse in a normal manner'. Little is known about this early version of a vacuum device, and the technique seems to have been forgotten until the 1960s when Geddings Osbon Sr developed the Erecaid, the first commercially available vacuum device designed to treat erectile dysfunction. Acceptance of this novel form of treatment came slowly. Mechanical devices designed to treat impotence had been largely ignored by the medical profession as they were thought to belong in back street sex shops; indeed, the US Post Office charged the manufacturers of the Erecaid with sending pornographic material by mail. Attitudes eventually changed, and in the early 1970s the Erecaid became the first vacuum device to be approved by the US Food and Drug Administration.

Mechanism of action

The mechanism of action of vacuum devices is probably straightforward. The low pressure around the penis and within the cylinder enhances the flow of blood into the sinusoids of the corpus cavernosum. The constriction band then prevents the outflow of blood, so tumescence is maintained. There is some experimental evidence to

Table 4.4 How to use a vacuum device

1. Read the instructions, watch the accompanying video and familiarise yourself with the operation of the device
2. Always use it with your partner in a situation where you would expect to have intercourse. It is less likely to work if you are not aroused
3. Apply lubricant generously around the penis, inside the cylinder and on the outside of the base of the cylinder (to facilitate removing the constriction ring)
4. Apply the constriction ring to the outside of the cylinder
5. Place the cylinder over the penis, press firmly against the body and operate the suction pump
6. If an adequate erection is obtained slip the constriction ring off the base of the cylinder so it is tight around the base of the penis and remove the cylinder
7. If the erection is inadequate at this stage reapply the cylinder and, with the constriction ring in place, operate the pump again
8. When intercourse is over, carefully remove the ring

support this assumption. It is difficult to measure penile blood flow during the application of a vacuum device. Broderick et al, using Duplex ultrasonography, reported that the low-pressure environment increased central cavernous arterial blood flow velocities.[17] Using blood gas analysis, it has been reported that in addition to increased arterial inflow, vacuum therapy also causes increased venous backflow.[18] Application of the constriction ring produces ischaemia, with little measurable blood-flow, which results in the penis feeling cold. It is reasonable to assume, however, that some blood flow must be maintained, as there have been very few reported cases of gangrene or auto-amputation of the penis with use of a vacuum device even though there have been anecdotal case reports of constriction rings being left on all night. The instructions of how to use a vacuum device are listed in Table 4.4.

Trial data

The nature of impotence treatment make undertaking controlled trials difficult. The choice of any particular treatment is a very personal one. An impotent man is much more likely to have an opinion on whether to use a vacuum device or self-injection therapy than he is on which antihypertensive agent to take. As a result, many trials of vacuum devices have allowed the patient to choose the treatment. Very few controlled trials have been done and, not surprisingly, none have been 'blinded'.

The early trials of vacuum devices were often done by enthusiastic investigators on selected patients at a time when other effective treatments for impotence were not readily available. It is therefore perhaps not surprising that the reported results were excellent and rather better than more recent experience would suggest. In one of the earliest trials of vacuum devices Nadig et al. reported that 32 out of 35 men with impotence of mixed aetiology were able to achieve an erection using an Erecaid and, subsequently, 24 used the device on a regular basis.[19] Several subsequent series of vacuum therapy in men with impotence of mixed aetiology have reported between 50% and 90% success.[20–26] None of these trials were controlled, but nonetheless the results left little doubt that vacuum devices were an effective treatment for impotence due to various aetiologies.

Results of trials of vacuum therapy in patients who had failed with self-injection treatment showed much lower success rates.[27,28] This is perhaps not surprising. Impotence treatments fail for a variety of reasons: many couples find any artificially induced erection unaccept-able, in other cases, there are relationship problems that no impotence treatment could overcome. Thus, any man whose impotence is not corrected with his first choice of treatment is less likely to have any success with another form of treatment.

Few studies have assessed the female partners' attitudes to vacuum devices. The limited data available suggest that this technique is as acceptable to women as it is to men.[29,30] In a study of 10 impotent diabetic men and their partners, Wiles reported 3 partners failed to come to terms with vacuum therapy but 6 found the technique acceptable.[16] Another study of the female partners of 9 impotent diabetic men reported high levels of partner satisfaction.[31] In this small study there were several positive benefits from the use of vacuum devices, including prolonged intercourse, the additional lubrication used and even the cold feeling of the penis!

Most trials of vacuum devices have been short term, few lasting longer than 6 months. In one of the few long-term studies of vacuum devices, Cookson and Nadig reported 70% of men were still using the device at 1 year.[32] In another study Turner et al. reported 80% of men were still using vacuum therapy at 1 year.[33] Overall, it would appear the long-term usage of vacuum therapy appears to be at least as good as self-injection therapy and probably better.

There has been little work published on why couples stop using vacuum devices. There is no evidence to suggest efficacy reduces or that the side effects worsen with time. Undoubtedly, many couples find the lack of spontaneity in using a vacuum device a problem. The advan-tages and disadvantages of vacuum devices are listed in Table 4.5.

Few studies examining the impact of vacuum therapy on self-esteem and well-being have been done. In a study of 29 men with impotence of mixed aetiology, Turner et al. reported no improvement

Table 4.5 Advantages and disadvantages of vacuum devices

Advantages

- Suitable for most men with erectile dysfunction, regardless of aetiology
- Side effects minor
- Few contraindications
- Suitable for frequent and long-term use
- Low cost

Disadvantages

- Erections can be uncomfortable
- Penis pivots at base
- Ejaculation can be impaired
- Lack of spontaneity
- Cumbersome
- Penis feels cold to partner

in psychological parameters despite good results in restoring inter-course.[30] In another study the same group found improvements in psychological functioning of both men and partners after 12 months' treatment with a vacuum device.[33]

Vacuum therapy in diabetic men

Trials in diabetic men with erectile dysfunction have shown results comparable with non-diabetic men, suggesting that it is an effective treatment in diabetes.[11,14–16] It would appear to be an effective treatment, regardless of the aetiology; good results have been reported in impotent diabetic men with extensive vascular disease or severe autonomic neuropathy.[11] In non-diabetic men, it appears to be effective if the erectile dysfunction is psychogenic in origin[34] or due to venous leakage.[11,35] In one remarkable study, vacuum therapy was effective in 16 out of 17 men in whom a penile implant had been removed. As this procedure causes considerable damage to the corpus cavernosum, it suggests vacuum devices require little functioning erectile tissue to be effective.[23]

Complications and contraindications

Vacuum therapy would appear to be a remarkably safe treatment for erectile dysfunction; very few serious adverse events have been reported. There has been one reported case of skin necrosis[36] following the use of a vacuum device and one case of penile gangrene.[37] Subcutaneous bruising is relatively common but is usually self-limiting. For this reason most manufacturers advise that bleeding diatheses or anticoagulation therapy are contraindications to the use of vacuum therapy.

Most other side effects are minor. Discomfort or pain due to the constriction band or during pumping is relatively common and can be the reason for discontinuing treatment. Failure to ejaculate can occur in up to one-third of men, but anorgasmia is rare.[16,19,20]

Which vacuum device?

At present there are more than six different vacuum devices on the market and there have been few attempts to compare them. The choice of vacuum device will depend on availability, price and personal preference. Details of suppliers can be obtained from the British Diabetic Association (see Appendix I).

Vacuum therapy versus injection therapy

The relative efficacy of one form of treatment for erectile dysfunction over another will depend on a variety of factors including patient preference. For this reason randomised trials are difficult to justify and not many have been done. One of the few trials suggested a preference for injection therapy over vacuum devices in a group of men with impotence of mixed aetiology.[38] In contrast, a non-randomised trial from Japan showed a clear preference for vacuum devices.[39] A meta-analysis of 209 publications on the treatment of erectile dysfunction showed comparable results for vacuum devices, papaverine and prostaglandin E_1 intracavernosal injection therapy, but vacuum therapy had the lowest drop-out rate.[40] Ultimately, what the individual patient thinks is the best treatment is more important than any published data.

Intracavernosal injection therapy

Introduction

In 1982 the French urologist Virag injected the vasodilator papaverine into the penis of a man undergoing penile surgery. History does not record why he did this but as the injection produced an erection he realised he had a potential treatment for impotence. He published this observation in a letter to the *Lancet*[41] and the idea was soon taken forward by others. Virag was not the first to try this technique; this distinction falls to Brindley who used phenoxybenzamine, but Virag won the race to publication.[42] Experience soon suggested papaverine was the more effective agent, and within a remarkably short space of time was widely used, alone or in combination with phentolamine, as a first line treatment for erectile dyfunction.[43–45]

Mechanism of action

Papaverine is a nonselective phosphodiesterase inhibitor which acts as a smooth muscle relaxant and vasodilator. When injected into the corpus cavernosum, it produces dilatation of the penile arteries and increases arterial inflow.[43] Cavernosography studies have also suggested injection of papaverine into the corpus cavernosum reduces venous outflow. Thus, papaverine may mimic the physiological changes that occur during tumescence when smooth muscle relaxation of the corpus cavernosum leads to compression of the venous sinusoids against the tunica albuginea and hence reduced venous outflow. The mechanism of action of prostaglandin E_1 is very similar (see below); however, the mode of action of phentolamine is rather different. It blocks adrenergically induced smooth muscle tone and therefore prolongs erection but does not initiate it.[46] As papaverine

acts at a late stage in the erection pathway, it is not very physiological in its action; therefore, its action does not depend on the man
being aroused, and if too much is given there is the risk of priapism.

Intracavernosal therapy in the treatment of impotence

The principle of self-injection therapy is fairly simple. Before intercourse the impotent man draws up the drug into a syringe, injects it
into the corpus cavernosum, massages the penis and waits until
tumescence occurs. Most early studies were done with papaverine,
which was rapidly adopted as the most widely used treatment for
erectile dysfunction across the world and was used by urologists,
diabetologists, psychiatrists and genitourinary physicians.[43,44,47,48]
Papaverine suffers from the disadvantage that it is an 'unphysiological'
method of inducing erections. In other words, it induces tumescence
regardless of whether the man is aroused and erections last until the
effects of the drug wear off; detumescence does not automatically
occur after ejaculation.

Alprostadil and papaverine: Results of clinical trials

Papaverine is not a licensed preparation and therefore there was no
support from the pharmaceutical industry to undertake controlled
clinical trials. As a result, most of the early work done on papaverine consisted of uncontrolled observations. However, the results of
early trials showed that papaverine was an effective treatment for
erectile dysfunction due to a variety of aetiologies.[44,45,47,48] In diabetic
men, Alexander reported that effective treatment for erectile dysfunction could be offered using papaverine self-injection with good
results.[13]

Alprostadil (prostaglandin E_1, Caverject, Pharmacia & Upjohn;
Viridal, Schwarz) became licensed for self-injection treatment of
erectile dysfunction in 1996 and has subsequently largely displaced
papaverine. Both agents are effective, but alprostadil has considerable
advantages, being a licensed product. It is packaged specifically for
self-injection treatment in a container with the necessary syringe,
needles and instructions. However, it suffers from the disadvantage

that it comes as a powder and separate solvent. These must be mixed immediately prior to injection, as the solution has a short shelf life. This has been made simpler by the introduction of dual-chamber injection devices that allow for easy mixing and dose adjustment (Fig. 4.1). The few controlled studies done comparing papaverine and alprostadil have suggested that alprostadil is as good or slightly better than papaverine in terms of efficacy and tolerability.[13,49,50]

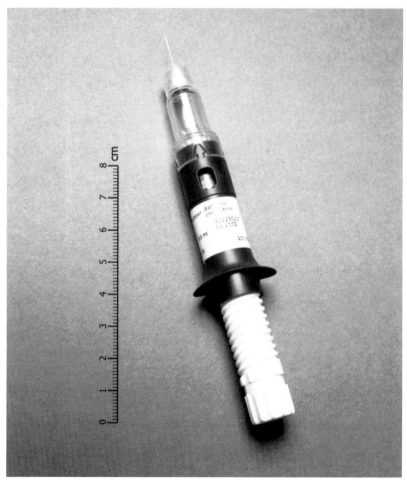

Figure 4.1 *Alprostadil self-injection device.*

In spite of all the problems associated with self-injection treatment, it rapidly became the most popular treatment for erectile dysfunction. A survey undertaken in 1996, before effective oral therapies became available, showed that it was the treatment of choice of 67% of diabetologists in the United Kingdom (O'Malley and Price, unpublished data).

Long-term data

One of the most disappointing aspects of self-injection therapy is the high long-term discontinuation rate. Most long-term studies of papaverine have reported that between 40 and 80% of couples give up using self-injection therapy.[51–54] Some of these studies have also addressed the question why couples stop using self-injection therapy. In most cases, couples stop using self-injection therapy because of loss of interest. It would appear that failure of treatment or adverse events are not major reasons for its discontinuation.[51,54]

Affects on quality of life measures

A few studies have attempted to examine the effects of treating impotence with self-injection treatment on quality of life measures. Althof et al. reported that the use of self-injection with papaverine and phentolamine produced improvements in general psychiatric symptomatology in the men but not their partners.[55] Willke et al. have reported in two studies that treatment of erectile dysfunction with alprostadil produced improvements in measures of mental health and overall quality of life.[56]

Complications of self-injection therapy

As self-injection therapy using papaverine was widely adopted as a treatment for erectile dysfunction, it soon became apparent that it was commonly associated with a number of complications. Of these, priapism – a sustained unwanted erection – is the most important.[57–59] A meta-analysis of 10 published studies suggested the median probability of priapism (per person) using papaverine was 0.093 (95%

confidence interval 0.049–0.156) and 0.031 (0.017–0.053) for alprostadil.[40] Thus, it is not a frequent complication but is clearly an important one. Any man contemplating self-injection treatment must be warned of this complication and given specific instruction as to what to do should it occur. Younger men with psychogenic or neurogenic impotence with better baseline erectile function appear to be at greater risk of developing priapism and those with vasculogenic impotence have the least risk.[58] However, no man treated with self-injection therapy is immune from the risk of priapism and so should be advised appropriately.

Should priapism occur, treatment must be prompt. If the erection persists for more than 2 hours then there are several manoeuvres that can be undertaken that may terminate the erection. It has been reported that vigorous leg exercises, such as peddling an exercise bicycle or running up and down stairs, can end an erection.[61] Any man using self-injection treatment must be warned to seek urgent medical advice should these manoeuvres fail and the erection persists for more than 6 hours. This is made considerably easier if he already has written instructions to take to the nearest hospital emergency department and show to the on-call physician, who may not be familiar with the correct procedure.

Local adverse reactions, such as penile pain, are relatively common. In the same meta-analysis described above, the probability of local pain or discomfort was reported to be 0.189 (0.101–0.303) with papaverine and 0.233 (0.175–0.304) with alprostadil.[40] This is slightly more than with vacuum devices.

Prolonged use of self-injection therapy may lead to fibrosis in the penis. This usually takes the form of painless nodules, but can be more extensive so as to obliterate the corpus cavernosum and preclude the insertion of a penile implant.[59,61,62] Because of the risk of fibrosis, it is generally advised that papaverine is not used more than once a week. Fibrosis has only rarely been reported with alprostadil self-injection therapy.[40]

Several other local adverse events have been reported with the use of self-injection therapy, including bone formation,[63] purulent cavernositis[64] and needle breakage.[65] However, for such a widely-used treatment, the likelihood of any of these problems occurring must be very small. Minor systemic problems can also occur with papaverine intracavernosal injection. Dizziness due to escape of papaverine into the systemic circulation has been reported but is rare.[66] Minor abnormalities of liver function tests are relatively common.[59]

Self-injection therapy in diabetic men

Few studies have been done examining the role of self-injection therapy specifically in diabetic men, but the available evidence suggests the results are little different to those in non-diabetics.[67] Alexander reported that it was perfectly feasible for a physician to offer treatment for erectile dysfunction within a diabetic clinic using self-injection therapy.[13]

Other injectable agents

Vasoactive intestinal polypeptide

Vasoactive intestinal polypeptide (VIP) is a vasodilator that has a role in the development of erection. When injected into the corpus cavernosum as a single agent it has only modest effects, producing a limp erection; however, when given in combination with phentolamine it appears to be a potentially useful treatment for erectile dysfunction.[68] In a study of men with erectile dyfunction of mixed aetiology the combination produced an erection sufficient for intercourse in all 52 men treated and at 6 months follow up over 80% of the men were still using the treatment.[69] In a more recent study the combination of VIP and phentolamine given by injection worked in 67% of men who had failed on other vasoactive agents.[70] At the time of writing there have been no studies published on this treatment in diabetic men.

The combination of VIP and phentolamine has been given the trade name Invicorp. It is administered in a preloaded spring-loaded self-injection device which is simple and easy to use but has yet to be released onto the market.

89

Transurethral alprostadil

Self-injection treatment suffers from the considerable disadvantage that it requires a needle to be inserted into the penis. There was considerable interest therefore when a transurethral preparation of alprostadil became available. The principle is quite simple: a slender applicator is inserted into the urethra to deposit a pellet containing alprostadil in polyethylene glycol (PEG). This gradually dissolves, allowing the prostaglandin to diffuse into the corpus cavernosum. This preparation has been marketed with the acronym MUSE (medicated urethral system for erection). The applicator is neat and simple to use (Fig. 4.2) and most men find it preferable to a needle. Transurethral alprostadil seems to have a success rate slightly less than the injectable preparation. Padma-Nathan et al. reported, in a placebo controlled study of 1511 men with erectile dysfunction of mixed aetiology, that 65% were able to have inter-course using MUSE.[71] The results in diabetic men were similar. The success rate amongst the 240 diabetic men in the study was 64.3%.[72] The most common side effect was penile pain, which occurred in 10.8% of alprostadil treatments. Hypotension was reported by 3.3% of men receiving alprostadil. Priapism and penile fibrosis were not reported.

Transurethral alprostadil is best administered after emptying the bladder to improve lubrication. After administration, the penis should be massaged to improve adsorption of the drug. There is then a delay of approximately 30 min during which time the man is advised to remain standing.

When given the choice, most men initially prefer transurethral alprostadil over self-injection treatment. However, the anecdotal experience of most clinicians is that transurethral alprostadil does not produce the same degree of penile rigidity as self-injection treatment and a comparative study of 111 men suggested intracavernosal injection therapy was more efficacious and better tolerated than MUSE and preferred by the patients.[73]

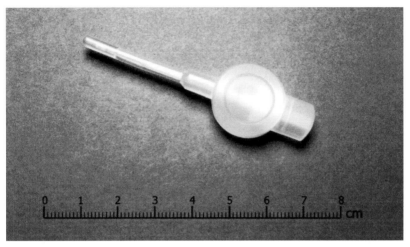

Figure 4.2 *Transurethral alprostadil (MUSE).*

Oral agents

Androgens

Testosterone therapy is indicated for the treatment of erectile dysfunction only in men with confirmed hypogonadism. Similarly, dopamine agonists should only be used in patients with hyperprolactinaemia. A diabetic man with hypogonadism and erectile dysfunction should be warned that testosterone therapy will probably restore libido but may not necessarily improve erectile function.

Yohimbine

Yohimbine is an agent long considered an aphrodisiac. It is derived from the bark of the yohimbe tree, which grows in Africa, and from the root of the rauwolfia tree which is found in Southeast Asia. It is an alpha$_2$ antagonist that acts both centrally and peripherally. It is not certain if its actions on erectile function derive from its central or peripheral actions. Published evidence on the efficacy of yohimbine in the treatment of erectile dysfunction is conflicting. In a study of 48 men with psychogenic impotence a 42% response rate was claimed.[74] The response rate in a study of 100 men with erectile dysfunction of organic origin was not significantly better than placebo.[75] A meta-analysis of 445 patients in four trials suggested yohimbine was of little benefit in organic impotence.[40] The efficacy of yohimbine in treating erectile dysfunction in diabetic men has not been reported. Many diabetologists have prescribed it and anecdotally it appears to be effective in a few patients, particularly if the erectile dysfunction is psychogenic in aetiology. However, it is not widely available and has not caught on as a treatment for impotence in diabetes.

Phentolamine

Phentolamine is an alpha$_1$- and alpha$_2$-receptor antagonist. It has been used in the past as an intracavernosal agent, but recently there has been a resurgence of interest in phentolamine as an oral treatment of impotence. Becker et al. reported a 50% response rate in a small group of men with organic impotence.[76] In a study of phentolamine given by buccal application, Zorgniotti et al. reported a 42% response in men with erectile dysfunction of mixed aetiology.[77] At the time of writing, an oral preparation of phentolamine under the trade name Vasomax is undergoing phase III clinical trials. Success rates of 55–59% have been reported in the treatment of erectile dysfunction in mixed groups of patients.[78] Oral phentolamine has also been reported to increase the success rates when used with intracavernosal alprostadil.[79]

Apomorphine

Apomorphine is a centrally acting D2 dopamine receptor antagonist. The exact role of the dopamine pathway in sexual function in humans is uncertain but it is likely that dopamine acts on neurons in the paraventncular nucleus of the hypothalamus and proerectile sacral parasympathetic nucleus in the spinal cord.[80] The potential role of apomorphine in the treatment of ED has been known for many years. More recently the availability of a fast acting sublingual preparation has given this compound a new lease of life. Heaton et al reported that sublingual apomorphine improved erections in 7 of 11 men with

ED of mixed aetiology. This preparation was licensed for the treatment of ED in Europe in 2001 and is being marketed by a major pharmaceutical company.

Overall sublingual apomorphine restores successful sexual intercourse in approximately 50% of men with ED of mixed aetiology.[82,83] It has the advantage of rapid onset of action, usually within 20 minutes. It is safe and generally well tolerated. Nausea, headache and dizziness occur in approximately 7% of cases. No studies of the efficacy of apomorphine in diabetic men have been published.

Trazodone

Trazodone is an antidepressant with alpha-blocking activity. It has been reported to occasionally cause priapism and is used empirically to treat erectile dysfunction. It has been suggested that trazodone can enhance penile erection by interfering with the sympathetic control of penile detumescence.[84] One controlled trial of trazodone has been reported. In a group of men with mainly psychogenic impotence it was no more effective than placebo.[85] It is unlikely that trazodone will have a significant role to play in the management of erectile dysfunction in diabetes.

Topical pharmacological treatment for erectile dysfunction

Most men would find it more acceptable to apply a cream or ointment on the penis rather than inject a drug into the corpus cavernosum. For this reason, several topical agents have been tried as treatments for erectile dysfunction. These include nitrates,[86] papaverine,[87] minoxidil[88,89] and prostaglandin E_1.[90] The results are not very impressive and none has stood the test of time.

Phosphodiesterase (PDE) 5 Inhibitors

Sildenafil

Background. In the early 1990s a potential new cardiovascular drug, UK 92,480, was undergoing phase I and II studies at Pfizer Central Research, Sandwich, Kent. Many of the men who took the new agent reported to the investigators that their previous erectile dysfunction had resolved. The drug was later given the name sildenafil (Viagra), and the decision was taken to investigate its potential as a treatment for erectile dysfunction. History does not record how effective it was as a cardiovascular drug but overnight the management of erectile dysfunction had been transformed.

Mechanism of action. Sildenafil is a selective inhibitor of phosphodiesterase type 5 (PDE 5), an enzyme found in smooth muscle, platelets and the corpus cavernosum. The mechanism of action is shown in Fig. 4.3. Under conditions of sexual stimulation there is an increase in the intracellular concentrations of nitric oxide, which acts via the second messenger cyclic guanosine monophosphate (cGMP) to produce smooth muscle relaxation (see above). This is broken down in turn by PDE 5. As sildenafil inhibits the actions of PDE V, it has the potential to enhance erections under conditions of sexual stimulation. Thus, in theory, sildenafil should only enhance the physiological process of erection, such as during sexual arousal. Support for this hypothesis comes from a study which reported that sildenafil enhances nocturnal erections.[91] Conversely, as the process of erection requires the presence of nitric oxide, sildenafil might not be expected to work in the absence of nitric oxide tone.

Evidence to support this mode of action of sildenafil comes from work done on human corpus cavernosal tissue in vitro. Sildenafil produced a dose-dependent increase in smooth muscle relaxation under conditions of electrical field stimulation. In contrast, field stimulation alone produced only modest relaxation.[92]

Clinical trial data. Initial clinical trials with sildenafil were very promising. The first study, in 12 men with erectile dysfunction of no known cause, measured efficacy using penile rigiscanning during visual sexual stimulation. Sildenafil was significantly superior to placebo.[93] A second similar study in diabetic men with erectile dysfunction showed sildenafil produced significant improvements in penile rigidity and sexual function.[94] Both these studies used a maximum dose of 50 mg. The pivotal study was published in 1998.

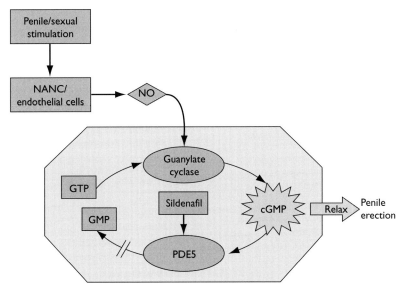

Figure 4.3 *Mechanism of action of sildenafil. cGMP, cyclic guanosine monophosphate; GTP, guanosine triphosphate; NANC, nonadrenergic noncholinergic; NO, nitric oxide; PDE5, phosphodiesterase V.*

Five hundred and thirty-two men with erectile dysfunction of mixed aetiology were studied. In the group given sildenafil, 69% of all attempts at intercourse were successful, compared with 22% in those given placebo.[95] Other studies in men with erectile dysfunction of mixed aetiology have shown similar results with success rates of between 65 and 77%.[96,97] Studies of sildenafil in other patient groups have reported success rates varying from 70% in men with hypertension,[98] 76% in spinal cord injury,[99] 63% in spina bifida,[100] 67% in men undergoing dialysis[101] and 40% following radical prostatectomy.[102]

In diabetic men the success rates for sildenafil have been reported to be between 56% and 59% in the treatment of erectile dysfunction.[50,98,103] Sildenafil has not been available long enough for any study of long-term usage, but in the experience of the author, of 7 diabetic men using sildenafil for 6 years none developed significant adverse events and there was no significant loss of efficacy, although one discontinued its use because of the need for nitrate therapy.

Predicting the response to sildenafil.   The reasons why up to 50% of men do not respond to sildenafil remain unclear. Jarow et al. examined factors predicting response in 267 men and reported that outcome was related to baseline sexual function but no single factor precluded success.[104]   Pegge et al.[105]   examined autonomic and endothelial function in diabetic and non-diabetic men with erectile dysfunction. They reported no difference in either parameter in sildenafil responders compared with non-responders.

Spontaneous return of function.   It is a commonly expressed view that, after successful treatment of impotence, erectile activity can return spontaneously to normal. This idea has a certain intellectual appeal. If the erectile dysfunction is due in part to performance anxiety, then restoring sexual function with a physical treatment might enable the man to overcome his fear of failure, allowing him to attempt intercourse with more confidence. However, there is only anecdotal evidence to back this up, and a review of the literature suggests that spontaneous return of function in a group of men with erectile dysfunction of mixed aetiology is no greater than the expected placebo response.[106] As erectile dysfunction in diabetes usually has a physical cause, any spontaneous return of function is probably even less likely. Therefore, when offering treatment to an impotent diabetic man it is probably wise to advise that natural erections will not return and treatment will be long term.

Adverse effects.   The adverse events from a sub-analysis of 10 trials of sildenafil in diabetic men are given in Table 4.6 (DE Price, unpublished data). Headache and flushing might be expected, as sildenafil is a vasodilator. The dyspepsia associated with sildenafil is usually mild and may be due to relaxation of the cardiac sphincter of the stomach. Abnormal vision is experienced by about 6% of men taking sildenafil; this may be because the drug has some activity against

Table 4.6 Adverse effects of sildenafil

Adverse event	Placebo (*n* = 274)	Sildenafil (*n* = 418)
Headache	3%	13%
Dyspepsia	0	11%
Flushing	1%	7%
Respiratory tract infection	4%	6%
Abnormal vision	0.4%	6%

phosphodiesterase VI, which is a retinal enzyme. There have been no reports of sildenafil causing any permanent effects on vision.

Sildenafil and cardiovascular disease. Within weeks of the launch of sildenafil, many adverse cardiovascular events – including myocardial infarction and death – were reported in association with the use of the drug. These received considerable media coverage, causing concern amongst patients and some doctors. The public reaction was such that, for the first time, the American Food and Drug Administration opened an internet web site solely on the subject of sildenafil to inform the public and to address some of their concerns. Following the concern about the safety of sildenafil, several studies have been undertaken to examine the cardiovascular effects of the drug. A study in 14 men with ischaemic heart disease reported that sildenafil produced a small reduction in pulmonary and systemic arterial pressures but had no effect on right atrial pressure, cardiac output or heart rate.[107] A post-hoc subanalysis of studies in men on antihypertensive agents suggested sildenafil produced a minor reduction in blood pressure of short duration.[108]

Adverse events associated with the use of sildenafil have been closely monitored by the regulatory authorities in the United States and Europe and all the available evidence does not suggest that sildenafil, or any other erectile dysfunction treatment, is associated with an increased risk of cardiovascular events.[109]

However, restoration of sexual activity may be associated with increased risk, and the issue of cardiovascular status should be addressed in all patients with erectile dysfunction.

Cardiovascular risk. Sexual activity is no more strenuous than many ordinary daily activities such as playing golf or walking a mile in 20 min; thus, the risk of restoring sexual function in men with cardiovascular disease is small but measurable. It has been estimated that the relative risk of myocardial infarction increases by a factor of 2.5 in the 2 hours after sexual activity in a patient without a cardiovascular history and threefold in a patient with a previous myocardial infarction.[110] It has been suggested that men requiring treatment for erectile dysfunction should be classified according to their cardiovascular risk: those with the highest risk should be referred for a specialist cardiac evaluation; those not falling into this category could effectively be treated for erectile dysfunction in primary care.[109]

Sildenafil and nitrates. Sildenafil is absolutely contraindicated in the presence of any form of nitrate therapy. Both agents act via the nitric oxide–cGMP pathway and the combination can produce profound hypotension. If a patient on nitrate therapy seeks treatment for erectile dysfunction, there are two possible options: He could be offered an alternative treatment such as injection therapy or a vacuum, or the nitrates could be stopped or changed for an alternative. In all but the most straightforward cases, the anti-anginal therapy should only be changed in consultation with a cardiologist. However, nitrates are a symptomatic treatment only and discontinuation has no prognostic implications, so that it should be possible in most men with ischaemic heart disease.

It has been suggested that a nitrate can be safely given 24 hours after a sildenafil dose and that a long-acting nitrate should be stopped 1 week before using sildenafil.[107]

How to use sildenafil
Sildenafil should be taken orally about 1 hour before sexual activity. This period can be shortened to 30 min if it is taken on an empty stomach. After the 1 hour period, there is a window of opportunity

of about 4 hours when sexual activity can take place. The recommended starting dose is 50 mg; however, most diabetic men require 100 mg. Patients should be warned that the drug will only work in conjunction with sexual stimulation.

Media reaction and political aspects

The advent of sildenafil was greeted with a reaction from the media that was unparalleled. No other drug or medical advance has ever had the same coverage from newspapers or television. Much of the coverage focused on the potential cost to health services of treating erectile dysfunction with this new agent. Few health services pay for erectile dysfunction treatment. Only Sweden offers full reimbursement. In the United Kingdom the arrival of sildenafil provoked a change in the law. For the first time doctors were prevented from prescribing a licensed drug on the National Health Service. Treatment for erectile dysfunction became available on the National Health Service only in certain conditions, which are listed in Table 4.7. If a man's impotence was due to another cause, he would have to pay for a private prescription.

Although the politicians may not consider erectile dysfunction treatment a priority, most patients do. It was reported in a survey of patients' perceptions of the importance of treating erectile dysfunction that most considered it as important as most complications of diabetes, except renal disease and blindness[111].

Other PDE 5 inhibitors

At the time of writing sildenafil is the only PDE 5 hibitor licensed for the treatment of ED. Its success has made it inevitable that other pharmaceutical companies would try and produce other PDE 5 inhibitors and several are underdevelopment.

Tadalafil

Tadalafil is a PDE 5 inhibitor structurally dissimilar to sildenafil. It has a longer half life (17 hours) which gives it the potential advantage that a single dose restore sexual function for 24 hours or longer. It is also more specific for PDE 5 than sildenafil with little activity

Table 4.7 Conditions for which treatment for erectile dysfunction can be prescribed on the National Health Service

- Diabetes
- Multiple sclerosis
- Spinal cord injury
- Prostate cancer
- Treatment for renal failure
- Radical pelvic surgery
- Single gene neurological disease
- Prostactectomy
- Poliomyelitis
- Spina bifida
- Parkinson's disease
- Severe pelvic injury

against PDE 6. This means its adverse effects do not include visual disturbance. However, the efficacy and side effect profile of the two drugs would appear to be very similar (unpublished data).

Vardenafil
Vardenafil is a PDE 5 inhibitor structurally very similar to sildenafil. Little has been published on this compound but it appears to be similar to sildenafil in efficacy and tolerability.

Summary

There are a wide range of treatments available for the management of erectile dysfunction in diabetes. All diabetes care services should offer a treatment programme for erectile dysfunction, particularly as recently introduced treatments are highly effective and easy to use.

References

1. Benet AE, Rehman J, Holcomb RG, Melman A. The correlation between the new RigiScan plus software and the final diagnosis in the evaluation of erectile dysfunction. J Urol 1996; 156(6):1947–50.

2. McCulloch DK, Young RJ, Prescott RJ et al. The natural history of impotence in diabetic men. Diabetologia 1984; 26(6):437–40.

3. McCulloch DK, Hosking DJ, Tobert A. A pragmatic approach to sexual dysfunction in diabetic men: psychosexual counselling. Diabet Med 1986; 3(5):485–9.

4. Meuleman EJ, Diemont WL. Investigation of erectile dysfunction. Diagnostic testing for vascular factors in erectile dysfunction. Urol Clin N Am 1995; 22(4):803–19.

5. Padma-Nathan H, Goldstein I, Krane RJ. Evaluation of the impotent patient. Sem Urol 1986; 4(4):225–32.

6. Whitehead ED, Klyde BJ, Zussman S, Salkin P. Diagnostic evaluation of impotence. Postgrad Med 1990; 88:123–36.

7. Buvat J, Buvat-Herbaut M, Dehaene JL, Lemaire A. Is intracavernous injection of papaverine a reliable screening test for vascular impotence? J Urol 1986; 135(3):476–8.

8. Bancroft J, Wu FC. Changes in erectile responsiveness during androgen replacement therapy. Arch Sex Behav 1983; 12(1):59–66.

9. Buvat J, Lemaire A. Endocrine screening in 1,022 men with erectile dysfunction: clinical significance and cost-effective strategy. J Urol 1997; 158(5):1764–7.

10. Hassan AA, Hassouna MM, Taketo T et al. The effect of diabetes on sexual behavior and reproductive tract function in male rats. J Urol 1993; 149(1):148–54.

11. Price DE, Cooksey G, Jehu D et al. The management of impotence in diabetic men by vacuum tumescence therapy. Diabet Med 1991; 8(10):964–7.

12. Masters WH, Johnson VE. Human Sexual Inadequacy. London: Churchill; 1970.

13. Alexander WD. The diabetes physician and an assessment and treatment programme for male erectile impotence. Diabet Med 1990; 7(6):540–3.

14. Bodansky HJ. Treatment of male erectile dysfunction using the active vacuum assist device. Diabet Med 1994; 11(4):410–12.

15. Ryder RE, Close CF, Moriarty KT et al. Impotence in diabetes: aetiology, implications for treatment and preferred vacuum device. Diabet Med 1992; 9(10):893–8.

16. Wiles PG. Successful non-invasive management of erectile impotence in diabetic men. Br Med J Clin Res Ed 1988; 296(6616):161–2.

17. Broderick GA, McGahan JP, Stone AR, White RD. The hemodynamics of vacuum constriction erections: assessment by color Doppler ultrasound. J Urol 1992; 147(1):57–61.

18. Bosshardt RJ, Farwerk R, Sikora R et al. Objective measurement of the effectiveness, therapeutic success and dynamic mechanisms of the vacuum device. Br J Urol 1995; 75(6):786–91.

19. Nadig PW, Ware JC, Blumoff R. Noninvasive device to produce and maintain an erection-like state. Urology 1986; 27(2):126–31.

20. Baltaci S, Aydos K, Kosar A, Anafarta K. Treating erectile dysfunction with a vacuum tumescence device: a retrospective analysis of acceptance and satisfaction. Br J Urol 1995; 76(6):757–60.

21. Cooper AJ. Preliminary experience with a vacuum constriction device (VCD) as a treatment for impotence. J Psychosom Res 1987; 31(3):413–18.

22. Korenman SG, Viosca SP, Kaiser FE et al. Use of a vacuum tumescence device in the management of impotence. J Am Geriatr Soc 1990; 38(3):217–20.

23. Korenman SG, Viosca SP. Use of a vacuum tumescence device in the management of impotence in men with a history of penile implant or severe pelvic disease. J Am Geriatr Soc 1992; 40(1):61–4.

24. Sidi AA, Lewis JH. Clinical trial of a simplified vacuum erection device for impotence treatment. Urology 1992; 39(6):526–8.

25. Vrijhof HJ, Delaere KP. Vacuum constriction devices in erectile dysfunction: acceptance and effectiveness in patients with impotence of organic or mixed aetiology. Br J Urol 1994; 74(1):102–5.

26. Witherington R. Vacuum constriction device for management of erectile impotence. J Urol 1989; 141(2):320–2.

27. Earle CM, Seah M, Coulden SE et al. The use of the vacuum erection device in the management of erectile impotence. Int J Impot Res 1996; 8(4):237–40.

28. Gilbert HW, Gingell JC. Vacuum constriction devices: second-line conservative treatment for impotence. Br J Urol 1992; 70(1):81–3.

29. Althof SE, Turner LA, Levine SB et al. Through the eyes of women: the sexual and psychological responses of women to their partner's treatment with self-injection or external vacuum therapy. J Urol 1992; 147(4):1024–7.

30. Turner LA, Althof SE, Levine SB et al. Treating erectile dysfunction with external vacuum devices: impact upon sexual, psychological and marital functioning. J Urol 1990; 144(1):79–82.

31. Maddison W, Roland JM. Vacuum tumescence: the female perspective. Diabet Med 1995; 12(10, supplement 2):S3.

32. Cookson MS, Nadig PW. Long-term results with vacuum constriction device. J Urol 1993; 149(2):290–4.

33. Turner LA, Althof SE, Levine SB et al. External vacuum devices in the treatment of erectile dysfunction: a one-year study of sexual and psychosocial impact. J Sex & Marital Ther 1991; 17(2):81–93.

34. Segenreich E, Israilov SR, Shmueli J, Servadio C. Vacuum therapy combined with psychotherapy for management of severe erectile dysfunction. Eur Urol 1995; 28(1):47–50.

35. Blackard CE, Borkon WD, Lima JS, Nelson J. Use of vacuum tumescence device for impotence secondary to venous leakage. Urology 1993; 41(3):225–30.
36. Kaye T, Guay AT. Re: Skin necrosis caused by use of negative pressure device for erectile impotence. J Urol 1991; 146(6):1618–19.
37. Rivas DA, Chancellor MB. Complications associated with the use of vacuum constriction devices for erectile dysfunction in the spinal cord injured population. J Am Paraplegia Soc 1994; 17(3):136–9.
38. Soderdahl DW, Thrasher JB, Hansberry KL. Intracavernosal drug-induced erection therapy versus external vacuum devices in the treatment of erectile dysfunction. Br J Urol 1997; 79(6):952–7.
39. Wada H, Sato Y, Suzuki N et al. A study on the erectile response with the vacuum constriction device compared with intracavernous injection of a vasoactive drug. [in Japanese]. Nippon Hinyokika Gakkai Zasshi – Jap J Urol 1995; 86(2):321–4.
40. Montague DK, Barada JH, Belker AM et al. Clinical Guidelines Panel on Erectile Dysfunction: Summary Report on the Treatment of Organic Erectile Dysfunction. J Urol 1996; 156:2007–11.
41. Virag R. Intracavernous injection of papaverine for erectile failure. Lancet 1982; 2(8304):938.
42. Brindley GS. Cavernosal alpha-blockade: a new technique for investigating and treating erectile impotence. Br J Psychiatry 1983; 143:332–7.
43. Virag R, Frydman D, Legman M, Virag H. Intracavernous injection of papaverine as a diagnostic and therapeutic method in erectile failure. Angiology 1984; 35(2):79–87.
44. Keogh EJ, Watters GR, Earle CM et al. Treatment of impotence by intrapenile injections. A comparison of papaverine versus papaverine and phentolamine: a double-blind, crossover trial. J Urol 1989; 142(3):726–8.
45. Turner LA, Althof SE, Levine SB et al. Self-injection of papaverine and phentolamine in the treatment of psychogenic impotence. J Sex & Marital Ther 1989; 15(3):163–76.
46. Azadzoi KM, Payton T, Krane RJ, Goldstein I. Effects of intracavernosal trazodone hydrochloride: animal and human studies. J Urol 1990; 144(5):1277–82.
47. Robinette MA, Moffat MJ. Intracorporal injection of papaverine and phentolamine in the management of impotence. Br J Urol 1986; 58(6):692–5.
48. Keogh EJ, Earle CM, Carati CJ et al. Treatment of impotence by intrapenile injections of papaverine and phenoxybenzamine: a double blind, controlled trial. Austral & NZ J Med 1989; 19(2):108–12.
49. Lee LM, Stevenson RW, Szasz G. Prostaglandin E1 versus phentolamine/papaverine for the treatment of erectile impotence: a double-blind comparison. J Urol 1989; 141(3):549–50.

50. Sarosdy MF, Hudnall CH, Erickson DR et al. A prospective double-blind trial of intracorporeal papaverine versus prostaglandin E1 in the treatment of impotence. J Urol 1989; 141(3):551–3.

51. Weiss JN, Badlani GH, Ravalli R, Brettschneider N. Reasons for high drop-out rate with self-injection therapy for impotence. Int J Impot Res 1994; 6(3):171–4.

52. Pagliarulo A, Ludovico GM, Cirillo-Marucco E et al. Compliance to longterm vasoactive intracavernous therapy. Int J Impot Res 1996; 8(2):63–4.

53. Flynn RJ, Williams G. Long-term follow-up of patients with erectile dysfunction commenced on self injection with intracavernosal papaverine with or without phentolamine. Br J Urol 1996; 78(4):628–31.

54. Armstrong DK, Convery AG, Dinsmore WW. Reasons for patient dropout from an intracavernous auto-injection programme for erectile dysfunction. Br J Urol 1994; 74(1):99–101.

55. Althof SE, Turner LA, Levine SB et al. Sexual, psychological, and marital impact of self-injection of papaverine and phentolamine: a long-term prospective study. J Sex & Marital Ther 1991; 17(2):101–12.

56. Willke RJ, Glick HA, McCarron TJ et al. Quality of life effects of alprostadil therapy for erectile dysfunction. J Urol 1997; 157(6):2124–8.

57. Padma-Nathan H, Goldstein I, Krane RJ. Treatment of prolonged or priapistic erections following intracavernosal papaverine therapy. Sem Urol 1986; 4(4):236–8.

58. Lomas GM, Jarow JP. Risk factors for papaverine-induced priapism. J Urol 1992; 147(5):1280–1.

59. Levine SB, Althof SE, Turner LA et al. Side effects of self-administration of intracavernous papaverine and phentolamine for the treatment of impotence. J Urol 1989; 141(1):54–7.

60. Alexander W. Detumescence by exercise bicycle. Lancet 1989; 1(8640):735.

61. Fuchs ME, Brawer MK. Papaverine-induced fibrosis of the corpus cavernosum. J Urol 1989; 141(1):125.

62. Desai KM, Gingell JC. Penile corporeal fibrosis complicating papaverine self-injection therapy for erectile impotence. Eur Urol 1988; 15(1–2):132–3.

63. Vapnek J, Lue TF. Heterotopic bone formation in the corpus cavernosum: a complication of papaverine-induced priapism. J Urol 1989; 142(5):1323–4.

64. Schwarzer JU, Hofmann R. Purulent corporeal cavernositis secondary to papaverine-induced priapism. J Urol 1991; 146(3):845–6.

65. Beer SJ, See WA. Intracorporeal needle breakage: an unusual complication of papaverine injection therapy for impotence. J Urol 1992; 147(1):148–50.

66. Wespes E, Schulman CC. Systemic complication of intracavernous papaverine injection in patients with venous leakage. Urology 1988; 31(2):114–15.

67. Tsai YS, Lin JS, Lin YM. Safety and efficacy of alprostadil sterile powder (S. Po., CAVERJECT) in diabetic patients with erectile dysfunction. Eur Urol 2000; 38(2):177–83.

68. Kiely EA, Bloom SR, Williams G. Penile response to vasoactive intestinal polypeptide alone and in combination with other vasoactive agents. Br J Urol 1989; 64:191–4.

69. Gerstenberg TC, Metz P, Ottesen B, Fahrenkrug J. Intracavernous self-injection with vasoactive intestinal polypeptide and phentolamine in the management of erectile failure. J Urol 1992; 147(5):1277–9.

70. Dinsmore WW, Alderdice DK. Vasoactive intestinal polypeptide and phentolamine mesylate administered by autoinjector in the treatment of patients with erectile dysfunction resistant to other intracavernosal agents. Br J Urol 1998; 81(3):437–40.

71. Padma-Nathan H, Hellstrom WJ, Kaiser FE et al. Treatment of men with erectile dysfunction with transurethral alprostadil. Medicated Urethral System for Erection (MUSE) Study Group. N Engl J Med 1997; 336(1):1–7.

72. Nolten WE, Billington CJ, Chiu KC et al. Treatment of erectile dysfunction (impotence) with a novel transurethral drug delivery system: results from a multicenter placebo-controlled trial [Abstract]. 10th International Congress of Endocrinology, 1996.

73. Shabsigh R, Padma-Nathan H, Gittleman M et al. Intracavernous alprostadil alfadex is more efficacious, better tolerated, and preferred over intraurethral alprostadil plus optional actis: a comparative, randomized, crossover, multicenter study. Urology 2000; 55(1):109–13.

74. Reid K, Surridge DH, Morales A et al. Double-blind trial of yohimbine in treatment of psychogenic impotence. Lancet 1987; 2(8556):421–3.

75. Morales A, Condra M, Owen JA et al. Is yohimbine effective in the treatment of organic impotence? Results of a controlled trial. J Urol 1987; 137(6):1168–72.

76. Becker AJ, Stief CG, Machtens S et al. Oral phentolamine as treatment for erectile dysfunction. J Urol 1998; 159(4):1214–6.

77. Zorgniotti AW. Experience with buccal phentolamine mesylate for impotence. Int J Impot Res 1994; 6(1):37–41.

78. Goldstein I. Oral phentolamine: an alpha-1, alpha-2 adrenergic antagonist for the treatment of erectile dysfunction. Int J Impot Res 2000; 12 (Suppl 1):S75–S80.

79. Kaplan SA, Reis RB, Kohn IJ et al. Combination therapy using oral alpha-blockers and intracavernosal injection in men with erectile dysfunction. Urology 1998; 52(5):739–43.

80. Heaton JP, Morales A, Adams MA, Johnston B, el-Rashidy R. Recovery of erectile function by the oral administration of apomorphine. Urology 1995; 45(2):200–6.

81. Giuliano F and Allard J. Dopamine and sexual function. International Journal of Impotence Research 2001; 13 (Suppl 3):S18–S28.

82. Morales A. Apomorphine to Uprima: the development of a practical erectogenic drug: a personal prospective. International Journal of Impotence Research 2001; 13 (Suppl 3): S29–S34.

83. Heaton JPW. Characterising the benefit of apomorphine SL (Uprima) as an optimised treatment for representative populations with erectile dysfunction. International Journal of Impotence Research 2001; 13 (Suppl 3): S35–S39.

84. Saenz de Tejada I, Ware JC, Blanco R et al. Pathophysiology of prolonged penile erection associated with trazodone use. J Urol 1991; 145(1):60–4.

85. Meinhardt W, Schmitz PI, Kropman RF, de la Fuente RB, Lycklama GA, Zwartendijk J. Trazodone, a double blind trial for treatment of erectile dysfunction. Int J Impot Res 1997; 9(3):163–5.

86. Owen JA, Saunders F, Harris C et al. Topical nitroglycerin: a potential treatment for impotence. J Urol 1989; 141(3):546–8.

87. Kim ED, el-Rashidy R, McVary KT. Papaverine topical gel for treatment of erectile dysfunction. J Urol 1995; 153(2):361–5.

88. Cavallini G. Minoxidil versus nitroglycerine: a prospective, double-blind, controlled trial in transcutaneous therapy for organic impotence. Int J Impot Res 1994; 6(4):205–12.

89. Chancellor MB, Rivas DA, Panzer DE et al. Prospective comparison of topical minoxidil to vacuum constriction device and intracorporeal papaverine injection in treatment of erectile dysfunction due to spinal cord injury. Urology 1994; 43(3):365–9.

90. Kim ED, McVary KT. Topical prostaglandin-E1 for the treatment of erectile dysfunction. J Urol 1995; 153(6):1828–30.

91. Montorsi F, Maga T, Strambi LF et al. Sildenafil taken at bedtime significantly increases nocturnal erections: results of a placebo-controlled study. Urology 2000; 56(6):906–11.

92. Ballard SA, Gingell CJ, Tang K et al. Effects of sildenafil on the relaxation of human corpus cavernosum tissue in vitro and on the activities of cyclic nucleotide phosphodiesterase isozymes. J Urol 1998; 159(6):2164–71.

93. Boolell M, Gepi-Attee S, Gingell JC, Allen MJ. Sildenafil, a novel effective oral therapy for male erectile dysfunction. Br J Urol 1996; 78(2):257–61.

94. Price DE, Gingell JC, Gepi-Attee S et al. Sildenafil: study of a novel oral treatment for erectile dysfunction in diabetic men. Diabet Med 1998; 15(10):821–5.

95. Goldstein I, Lue TF, Padma-Nathan H et al. Oral sildenafil in the treatment of erectile dysfunction. Sildenafil Study Group. N Engl J Med 1998; 338(20):1397–404.

96. Marks LS, Duda C, Dorey FJ et al. Treatment of erectile dysfunction with sildenafil. Urology 1999; 53(1):19–24.

97. Padma-Nathan H, Steers WD, Wicker PA. Efficacy and safety of oral sildenafil in the treatment of erectile dysfunction: a double-blind, placebo-controlled study of 329 patients. Sildenafil Study Group. Int J Clin Pract 1998; 52(6):375–9.
98. Price DE. Sildenafil citrate (Viagra) efficacy in the treatment of erectile dysfunction in patients with common concomitant conditions. Int J Clin Pract 1999; Supplement 102:21–3.
99. Giuliano F, Hultling C, El Masry WS et al. Randomized trial of sildenafil for the treatment of erectile dysfunction in spinal cord injury. Sildenafil Study Group. Ann Neurol 1999; 46(1):15–21.
100. Palmer JS, Kaplan WE, Firlit CF. Erectile dysfunction in patients with spina bifida is a treatable condition. J Urol 2000; 164(3 Pt 2):958–61.
101. Rosas SE, Wasserstein A, Kobrin S, Feldman HI. Preliminary observations of sildenafil treatment for erectile dysfunction in dialysis patients. Am J Kidney Dis 2001; 37(1):134–7.
102. Lowentritt BH, Scardino PT, Miles BJ et al. Sildenafil citrate after radical retropubic prostatectomy. J Urol 1999; 162(5):1614–17.
103. Rendell MS, Rajfer J, Wicker PA, Smith MD. Sildenafil for treatment of erectile dysfunction in men with diabetes: a randomized controlled trial. Sildenafil Diabetes Study Group. JAMA 1999; 281(5):421–6.
104. Jarow JP, Burnett AL, Geringer AM. Clinical efficacy of sildenafil citrate based on etiology and response to prior treatment. J Urol 1999; 162:722–5.
105. Pegge N, Twomey M, Ramsey M et al. Autonomic and endothelial function are impaired in erectile dysfunction but do not predict response to sildenafil. Diabet Med 2001; 18:89.
106. Sharlip ID. Does natural erectile function improve following intracavernous injections of vasoactive drugs? Int J Impot Res 1997; 9(4):193–6.
107. Herrmann HC, Chang G, Klugherz BD, Mahoney PD. Hemodynamic effects of sildenafil in men with severe coronary artery disease. N Engl J Med 2000; 342(22):1622–6.
108. Zusman RM, Prisant LM, Brown MJ. Effect of sildenafil citrate on blood pressure and heart rate in men with erectile dysfunction taking concomitant antihypertensive medication. Sildenafil Study Group. J Hypertens 2000; 18(12):1865–9.
109. Jackson G, Betteridge J, Dean J et al. A systematic approach to erectile dysfunction in the cardiovascular patient: a consensus statement. Int J Clin Pract 1999; 53(6):445–51.
110. Muller JE, Mittleman A, Maclure M et al. Triggering myocardial infarction by sexual activity. Low absolute risk and prevention by regular physical exertion. Determinants of Myocardial Infarction Onset Study Investigators. JAMA 1996; 275(18):1405–9.
111. Price DE, Rance J, Warehank et al. How much of a priority is treating erectile dysfunction? A study of patient's perception. Diabet Med 2001; 18:31.

chapter 5

The surgical treatment of erectile dysfunction in the diabetic patient

Clive Gingell

The surgical treatment of erectile dysfunction (ED) is usually reserved for those patients in whom more conservative methods have failed. In this respect, the diabetic patient is no different from any other man with organic erectile dysfunction who has failed to respond to or dislikes the less-invasive options of self-injection therapy and vacuum devices. The surgical options available are:

1. The insertion of penile prostheses
2. Corrective surgery for associated Peyronie's disease or post-injection corporal fibrosis
3. Venous and arterial surgery.

Penile prosthesis implantation

Preoperative counselling
It is extremely important that both the patient and, whenever possible, the partner are involved in the discussion regarding the different

prostheses available. No single prosthesis is best for every patient and the advantages and disadvantages need to be discussed. The wishes of the patient or couple are very important factors in device selection.

The cost of the prosthesis is an extremely important factor, particularly for treatment in the UK under the National Health Service, as many hospital trusts will not pay for the insertion of the considerably more expensive inflatable prostheses. Prosthesis implantation is an invasive form of therapy and patients must be warned regarding postoperative pain or discomfort, infection and the potential for reoperation, particularly if the inflatable prostheses are used. Post-operative pain, although variable, can be quite severe for several weeks after surgery and patients will need to restrict physical activity and coitus cannot be resumed for at least 4 and usually 6 weeks postoperatively. The complications of infection and possible erosion need to be discussed and that either of these complications usually require device removal. The patient also needs to be made aware that prostheses can fail mechanically and require reoperation. It is very important that the patient and his partner are made aware that the erection produced by a prosthesis is different from a normal erection, and this depends very much upon the type of prosthesis chosen. It is useful to show the patients examples of the prostheses and describe how they are inserted and the mechanism of action.

Preoperative preparation

Preoperative preparation is mainly directed at reducing the risk of infection and, in diabetic implant recipients, good control of diabetes mellitus may reduce the risk of infection. There is conflicting evidence as to whether diabetic men are at greater risk than non-diabetics for incurring infection following prosthesis implantation. Some studies suggest an increased risk,[1-3] whereas others report no evidence of increased risk.[4-6] There is a general agreement, however, that infectious complications which occur in diabetics are potentially more serious. In 1992 Bishop et al. reported that preoperative elevated glycosylated haemoglobin values (11.5% or higher) may correlate with an increased incidence of prosthesis infection in diabetic men.[7] Although in a recent large prospective study of 389 patients – including 114 diabetics – who underwent three–piece penile prosthesis implantation, no increased risk of infection was noted with increased levels of glycosylated haemoglobin. Prosthesis infections were commoner in diabetics, however (8.7% vs. 4.0%).[8] It would seem sensible, nevertheless, to ensure that the potential recipient of an implant has his diabetes under as good a control as possible before surgery.

Broad-spectrum antibiotics that provide cover against both Gram-negative and Gram-positive organisms should be given prophylactically and continued for at least 48 hours postoperatively; many surgeons prefer to continue oral medication for 1 week. The operative site is shaved in theatre and a prolonged and thorough skin preparation performed. Surgery should be deferred if there is any infective cutaneous lesion or dermatitis in the groins and, particularly in the uncircumcised diabetic, any balanitis.

Surgical approach
Implantation of penile prostheses can be performed through a variety of surgical approaches. The most commonly used are infrapubic, subcoronal and penoscrotal, the choice depending on the preference of the surgeon and the type of prosthesis to be implanted. Other considerations are related to any anatomical variations, corporal fibrosis and previous penile or pelvic surgery. The operation can be performed under general or regional anaesthesia, with some support for local anaesthesia on a day case basis.

Type of penile prosthesis
Surgically implantable penile prostheses are classified as either malleable or inflatable: many types are widely available and both classes have been improved significantly in recent years. Implants provide sufficient penile rigidity for sexual intercourse, and the type of prosthesis selected is dependent upon careful preoperative assessment and discussion with the patient and his partner.

The malleable prosthesis

A variety of semirigid rod penile prostheses of different designs are currently available (Figs 5.1 and 5.2). The most commonly available prostheses provide rigidity and flexibility by a core of braided silver

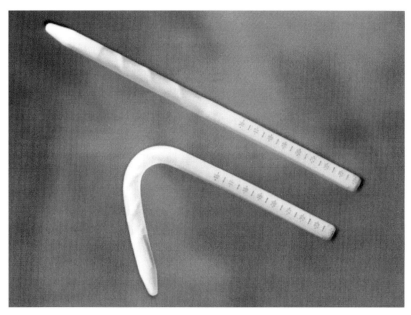

Figure 5.1 *The Acu-form malleable penile prosthesis. (Courtesy of Mentor Corporation.) This is trimmed in length at the time of surgery.*

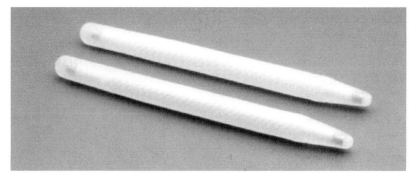

Figure 5.2 *The AMS malleable 650 penile prosthesis. The length is adjusted at surgery by the addition of rear tip extenders. (Courtesy of American Medical Systems, Inc.)*

wire running down the centre of a Silastic rod. The prosthesis and, hence, the penis, can be bent, and retains its position, allowing adjustment for intercourse or micturition. The disadvantage of such a prosthesis is that the penis is always in an erection-like state. With careful preoperative counselling and patient selection, patient and partner satisfaction is encouragingly good.[9] Concealment is often thought to be a major disadvantage with a malleable implant. However, 70% of patients in this study did not consider it to be a problem.

Malleable prostheses are considerably cheaper and quicker to insert than inflatable ones and they are particularly suitable for insertion under local anaesthesia on an outpatient or day case basis. For the maturity-onset diabetic with vasculogenic erectile failure, malleable prostheses are particularly appropriate and the short operative time minimises the risk of infection. Diabetic men are the most common organic group to require penile prosthetic surgery, this is an important consideration.

Inflatable penile prostheses
Modern multicomponent inflatable prostheses are now much more robust and reliable and are the most physiological prostheses available. They consist of an inflate/deflate pump placed in the scrotum, a storage reservoir placed retroperitoneally alongside the bladder and paired inflatable cylinders that are inserted into the corpora (Figs 5.3 and 5.4). The latter are inflated when required by the patient, who simply squeezes the small pump mechanism sited in the scrotum, and the penis can be returned to its dependent position by emptying the cylinders back into the small buried suprapubic reservoir by squeezing the deflate segment of the intrascrotal pump. The results with the inflatable penile prostheses are excellent and compare favourably with those reported for the more simple paired semirigid rods.

Postoperative management and complications
Adequate analgesia is required for pain relief in the early postoperative period. The discomfort can continue for several weeks and requires sympathetic management. Oral broad-spectrum antibiotics are required for 1 week after surgery, particularly in diabetes.

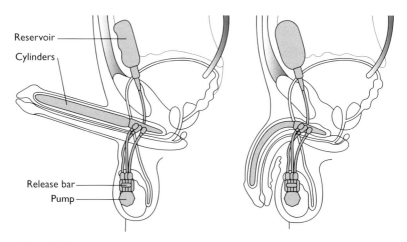

Figure 5.3 *Diagramatic illustration of the Mentor Alpha I inflatable penile prosthesis.*

Patients without voiding difficulties preoperatively rarely have a problem afterwards. Those that do, may require temporary catheterization. Infection is the most serious and significant complication of penile implant surgery, requiring reoperation and, frequently, removal of the device. The overall incidence of infection associated with penile prostheses is of the order of 2%, but it can be much higher. The introduction of an infection with *Staphylococcus epidermidis* at the time of implantation may induce a subclinical state of infection, causing chronic pain.[10] The importance of perioperative antibiotics, intraoperative shave and scrub, together with a strict surgical technique, is emphasised in a review by Radomski and Herschorn 1992,[11] resulting in a low prosthesis infection rate of 1.9%. They identified a group of patients who are at particular risk for infection, and this included diabetes. Another study by Lynch et al.[12] drew attention to the importance of a strict protocol, which significantly reduced the infection rate from 12.2% to 1.6%.

Patient and partner satisfaction

Many studies have assessed the outcome and degree of postoperative satisfaction of patients undergoing penile prosthesis implantation.

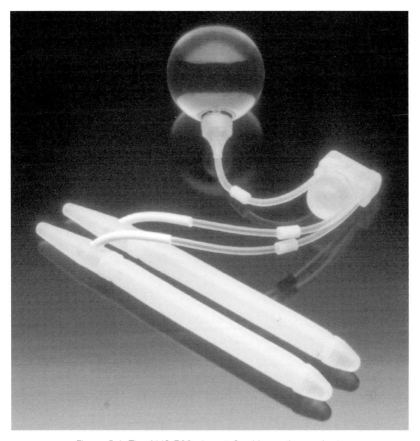

Figure 5.4 *The AMS 700 ultrex inflatable penile prosthesis.*

They have mainly been retrospective, however. Generally, they indicate a reasonable level of satisfaction, although the rates are less than surgical success rates. Clearly, the success of surgical treatment is closely linked to the patient and partner expectations. In the report on the treatment of organic erectile dysfunction developed by the Erectile Dysfunction Clinical Guidelines Panel of the American Urological Association Inc., published in 1996, the Outcome Balance Sheet Table for prostheses shows a range of estimated probabilities for patient satisfaction with various types of devices. This was 83.3% for

115

malleable prostheses and 88.9% for multicomponent inflatable devices. In 1994, a satisfaction study of the Alpha 1 prosthesis by Garber 1994[13] reported a 98% rate of satisfaction for 50 men followed from 2 to 41 months (average of 13 months).

Conclusions

Diabetic men are among the commonest patients that require penile prosthetic surgery and meticulous attention to detail is required to achieve a successful outcome. Careful preoperative counselling and patient selection will result in a very acceptable and durable end result. The malleable prostheses are very useful for the type II diabetic, who no longer participates in sporting activities that require communal showering. The young active diabetic patient with young or teenage children, who participates in swimming or other sporting events, requires the cosmetically more acceptable inflatable prostheses, in spite of the considerable increase in cost.

Peyronie's disease

Diabetic men have an increased incidence of Peyronie's disease (Fig. 5.5). Apart from the resultant penile curvature on erection associated with Peyronie's disease, many patients also have erectile dysfunction due to poor quality or poorly maintained erections, distal flaccidity and venous leakage.

Although conservative nonoperative treatment options are required in the early stages of the disease, until the pain and curvature settles, surgery may be indicated when the problem has stabilised. The usefulness of surgery in Peyronie's disease is well defined. If the patient is unable to penetrate because of curvature of the penis, then it may be straightened. In the Nesbit procedure, single or multiple ellipses or diamond-shaped segments of normal tunica albuginea are excised from the corpora cavernosa opposite the point of maximum curvature. Suturing then straightens the penis, albeit at the expense of length.[14,15] This operation is much simpler

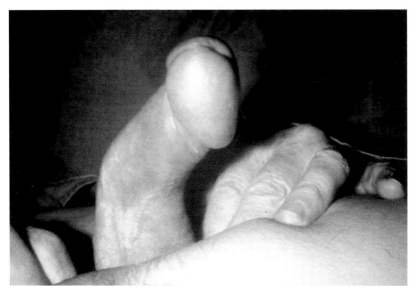

Figure 5.5 *Erect penis in a diabetic patient with Peyronie's disease, showing dorsal angulation.*

and less time-consuming than attempts at excising the plaque and replacing the defect with a dermal graft or other substitutes.[16] If the patient, in addition, has erectile failure that does not respond to intracavernosal injections, then the insertion of penile prostheses with or without incision of the plaques is a very effective procedure, which not only restores rigidity but also straightens the penis without any loss of length. With careful patient selection, surgical treatment should always restore sexual function.

Venous and arterial surgery

Venous leak surgery
Surgical procedures to correct venous incompetence are designed to correct corporovenous occlusive dysfunction by increasing the venous outflow resistance in the sinusoidal spaces of the corpora by

surgical resection of the deep dorsal vein of the penis and suture ligation of the circumflex veins draining into it.

After assessing the adequacy of arterial inflow to the penis by colour duplex scanning of the cavernosal arteries, patients are evaluated by using dynamic pharmacocavernosometry and cavernosography. Patients with veno-occlusive dysfunction typically complain of less than full quality erections which are poorly maintained and are not improved with the injection of intracorporeal vasoactive agents. The outcome of surgical intervention to correct erectile dysfunction due to venous leak have not been durable and failure rates have been high, despite appropriate selection.[17,18] Many patients, however, who previously did not respond positively to intracavernous injections have become responders after venous surgery. It is therefore worth considering investigating for a venous leak in younger patients who have not responded to oral or intracavernous therapy.

Arterial surgery

Arterial revascularization procedures have a very limited role in the treatment of erectile dysfunction in the diabetic, although they are effective in patients with pure arteriogenic erectile dysfunction caused by pelvic or perineal trauma.[19] Arterial revascularization is usually achieved using the inferior epigastric artery as the donor vessel with a variety of procedures incorporating the deep dorsal vein and dorsal arteries. As many diabetics have peripheral vascular disease, they are not usually candidates for this type of surgery and would be better served by the insertion of penile prostheses.

References

1. Kaufman JJ, Linder A, Raz S. Complications of penile prosthesis surgery for impotence. J Urol 1982; 128:1192–4.
2. Small MP. Small-carrion penile prosthesis: a report on 160 cases and review of the literature. J Urol 1978; 119:365–8.
3. Wilson SM, Wahman GE, Lange JL. Eleven years of experience with the inflatable prosthesis. J Urol 1988; 139:951-2.

4. Kabalin JN, Kessler R. Infectious complications of penile prosthesis surgery. J Urol 1988b; 139:953–5.
5. Montague DK. Periprosthetic infections. J Urol 1987; 138:68–9.
6. Thomalla JV, Thompson ST, Rowland RG et al. Infectious complications of penile prosthetic implants. J Urol 1987; 138:65–7.
7. Bishop JR, Moul JW, Sihelnik SA et al. Use of glycosylated haemoglobin to identify diabetics at high risk for penile periprosthetic infections. J Urol 1992; 147:386–8.
8. Wilson SK, Carson CC, Cleves MA, Delk II JR. Quantifying risk of penile prosthesis infection with elevated glycosylated haemoglobin. J Urol 1998; 159:1540.
9. Burns-Cox N, Burston A, Gingell JC. Fifteen years experience of penile prosthesis insertion. Int J Impot Res 1997; 9:211-216.
10. Parsons CL, Stein PC, Dobke MK et al. Diagnosis and therapy of subclinically infected prostheses. Surg Gynaeocol Obstet 1993; 177:504–6.
11. Radomski SB, Herschorn S. Risk factors associated with penile prosthesis infection. J Urol 1992; 147:383–5.
12. Lynch MJ, Scott GM, Inglis JA et al. Reducing the loss of implants following penile prosthetic surgery. Br J Urol 1994; 73:423–7.
13. Garber BB. Mentor Alpha 1 inflatable penile prosthesis: patient satisfaction and device reliability. Urology 1994; 43:214–17.
14. Nesbit RM. Congenital curvature of the phallus; a report of three cases with descriptions of corrective operation. J Urol 1965; 93:230–2
15. Pryor JP, Fitzpatrick JM. A new approach to the correction of the penile deformity in Peyronie's disease. J Urol 1979; 122:622–3.
16. Devine CJ, Horton CE. Surgical treatment of Peyronie's disease with a dermal graft. J Urol 1974; 111:44–9.
17. Freedman AL, Costa Neto F, Mehringer CM et al. Long term results of penile vein ligation for impotence from venous leakage. J Urol 1993; 149:1301-3.
18. Lue TF, Donatucci CF. Dysfunction of the veno-occlusive mechanism. In: Bennett AH, ed. Impotence. Diagnosis and Management of Erectile Dysfunction. Philadelphia: W.B. Saunders, 1994: 197–204.
19. Sharlip ID. Vasculogenic impotence secondary to atherosclerosis/dysplasia. In: Bennett AH, ed. Impotence. Diagnosis and Management of Erectile Dysfunction. Philadelphia: W.B. Saunders, 1994: 205–12.

chapter 6

How to organise an impotence clinic

William D Alexander

Introduction

Developing and providing a service for men with diabetes and erectile dysfunction can be both interesting and rewarding. It will, however, be time-consuming and require agreement with other clinicians and managers. It will also require initial training and ongoing personal education and development.

The service should be organised and run by someone with an interest in the management of erectile dysfunction. It requires the development of new skills and an ongoing requirement to keep apace of development. The mainstays of treatment are medical, well within the skills of most diabetology teams, and only a small minority of patients will require surgical intervention. Many associated psychological problems can be dealt with by the interested physician without the need for formal referral to psychological services. It is important, however, to establish and maintain links with other specialties including psychology and urology.

Models of clinics

Historically, a variety of different specialties have developed services for the management of erectile dysfunction. As a result, there are a variety of potential clinic structures and processes. These may involve physicians or surgeons working on their own or in multidisciplinary teams. Physicians and surgeons may also work with a specialist nurse or nurse practitioner who will usually do the practical training and reviews. General practitioners (GPs) can also manage erectile dysfunction, either for patients from their own practices or providing a service for a group of practices (see Chapter 7).

Initially, the erectile dysfunction clinic should probably be run by a consultant diabetologist, as it is important that the person leading the service is aware of and capable of managing the service they supervise. Once an erectile dysfunction clinic is established however, much of the work can effectively be done by clinical assistants and suitably trained nurses.

The clinic structure

In order to organise and set up a clinic it may be useful to consider the dynamics of it as a clinical service. What happens and what do you or your team have to have and have to do at each stage?

Patients are referred or identified

Patients will be identified either by self-presentation or by referral from another health care professional such as a specialist nurse, a GP or a colleague in another hospital specialty. A diabetologist must decide whether to see all impotent patients or just those with diabetes. It may be wise to start with the latter and see how large the caseload becomes and how much in the way of the clinic's and staff resources are forthcoming. It may be that, having initially established a service for diabetic patients, demands will come from other sources.

Patient numbers from the diabetic population will vary according to how hard you look. Screening the entire at-risk population of men is likely to produce a prevalence of up to 50%. It therefore may be sensible to initially use an awareness programme rather than screening. This can be done by the use of posters and leaflets in the clinic.

Clinicians undertaking *screening* for erectile dysfunction should be prepared to discuss the problem in general terms and make explanatory leaflets available to patients rather than just refer them on to another service. This is helpful to men and may prevent a number of unnecessary referrals as well as being educational and rewarding for the screeners.

Booking appointments

A clinic separate from the main diabetes clinic with dedicated appointments is preferable to an ad hoc service. It may be that the clinic can be managed within current resources. It is often easier to obtain resources for a service that is up and successfully running rather than for starting something new, and if you can start within your current resources this may be better.

New patients may take up to 1 hour if assessment and treatment are to be implemented in a single session, which includes instruction on self-injection therapy (Table 6.1).

The suggested times in Table 6.1 are based on you doing everything yourself and will also vary according to the amount of help available to you. Many clinics will run with the doctor doing the

Table 6.1 Times of assessment

Allow approximately the following time:

- History and examination: 15 min (this may be less for patients known to the diabetes clinic)
- General discussion about erectile dysfunction; discussion and explanation of practical aspects of various treatments, 15 min
- Instruction on intracorporeal injection therapy, 20 min
- Completing patient instruction sheets and GP letter, 10 min

Total = 60 min (with experience and *if* all goes really smoothly 30–40 min is possible)

assessment and discussion and a trained assistant instructing on the chosen treatment.

It may be preferred to separate treatment initiation from assessment to give men more time to think about the options and discuss them further with their partners. It is helpful, but should not be made mandatory, for men to bring their partners to the clinic but in the experience of most diabetologists less than 20% do so on the first occasion.

Follow-up appointments (unless requiring initial practical instruction) should be 10–15 min. Structure the clinic appointment template according to the times given in Table 6.1 and the method of running.

Some practitioners like to send men a questionnaire to be completed prior to the appointment and brought with them. There are a number of examples of such questionnaires. One standard and reasonably simple one is the International Index of Erectile Function (IIEF) questionnaire (Appendix I).

It can also be useful to send men information leaflets about erectile dysfunction with the appointment, so that they are reasonably informed when first seen. Despite the considerable publicity about erectile failure, many men remain unaware of the statistics and treatment possibilities.

Appointment letters and clinic directions should be discrete and marked 'Private and Confidential', because most men, at least initially, may be rather embarrassed about the problem.

The clinic venue

Facilities available will vary. A diabetes centre is ideal, as there will not be competition with other specialties for clinic space. Patients will know where it is and not therefore have the embarrassment of having to ask for directions and often hand over the appointment letter to a stranger in the corridor. It should be a nominated specialty clinic separate from diabetes review clinics. Clinics may be preferred 'out of hours' but it should be remembered that booking return appointments may be difficult unless administrative staff are available at the time. A video lounge may be useful for viewing educational videos but is not essential as patients can be lent videos to view at home.

A comfortable, relaxed and confidential atmosphere is important. Space is required for the clinician and the two partners as a minimum. There also needs to be storage space for equipment, videos, treatment demonstration, etc. An examination couch and wash basin are essential. A secure medicine cupboard should be available for the storage of drugs that may be used in the clinic. A refrigerator is also necessary for the storage of some drugs.

The clinical consultation

There is nothing unique about a clinical assessment for erectile failure. The process will be the same as for any presenting clinical problem. It will consist of a history, an examination and investigations, followed by discussion of treatment options and their implementation.

It may be found helpful to devise a proforma for use in the consultation. This can be helpful not only as a prompt but also for later audit purposes and registration on a computer database (see Appendix II). Table 6.2 lists some essential clinical aids for use during the consultation.

Table 6.2 Patient aids required in a clinic consultation

- Clerking proforma
- Intracavernosal injection kit for demonstration purposes
- Vacuum device for demonstration purposes
- Transurethral device (MUSE) for demonstration purposes
- Model penis
- Patient information leaflets
- Instructions regarding prolonged erections
- Instructions regarding doses for intracorporeal therapy (and other therapies)
- GP letter regarding prescribing and follow-up
- Instruction videos

Discussing and providing physical treatments

In many clinics this will now be done by a suitably trained nurse. At this stage it is worthwhile briefly mentioning all the treatments that are available and not only discussing these but, where appropriate, showing men examples of what, in principle, they would involve. Samples are easily available by request from the manufacturers or distributors. *It is worth having available:*

1. a model penis and a disposable insulin syringe to demonstrate the method of intracavernosal injection treatment, not necessarily the product that would actually be used, which will come later if appropriate
2. an example vacuum device
3. a sample introducer for transurethral treatment.
4. vacuum device order forms
5. educational leaflets

Oral or topically applied treatments

Explain the mode of action, potential side effects and warnings as appropriate, and advise on how to obtain prescriptions. It may be that treatments will seem initially ineffective. They must be given an adequate trial and used with associated sexual stimulation to ensure best results.

Vacuum devices

When discussing vacuum devices it is helpful to show men a device and the principle of how it works. Complications and unwanted effects should be explained. Many men will laugh and be inhibited at first sight, but it is worth persevering and explaining that men in stable and understanding relationships manage well with them. It is probably also worth giving all men an order form in case they later decide to consider this form of treatment. Cost should be mentioned. It may be possible to arrange for provision of some vacuum devices from the hospital appliance department and this is worth trying to negotiate.

Transurethral treatment

The principle of this form of treatment should be explained. Men who choose it should be shown the technique in detail and given an instruction leaflet or video. It is essential that the instructions are carefully adhered to in order to try and maximise absorption and reduce discomfort. Potential unwanted effects should be discussed.

Intracavernosal injection therapy

This is one of the most effective therapies and was one of the mainstays of treatment before the advent of oral therapies. Although it may be time-consuming, it should be demonstrated. It can be implemented during the initial consultation or alternatively a further appointment can be arranged.

Men may initially be reluctant to consider injecting their penis, even if they have previously been using insulin injections for diabetes control. However, men who do use intracorporeal injections are usually impressed at the simplicity of the procedure and, with good technique, that it is virtually painless. Overcoming potential needle shyness is therefore important, or many men may deny themselves an effective treatment because of false perceptions. This is a similar situation to starting anyone with diabetes on insulin therapy. It is important that men have at least actually seen or tried the treatment technique and know what it would entail before rejecting it. Two methods can be employed:

1. After demonstrating the technique using a model penis, you should explain that most men in your experience are astounded at how simple and painless it is and, using a plastic insulin syringe/needle, give a demonstration injection into the man's penis without actually injecting any drug. This is usually reassuring and can be followed by detailed instructions as in point 2 below.
2. If men have shown an interest in injection therapy you might say: 'Let me show you what injection treatment would involve.' Then get the man to mix and draw up the injection preparation as per the instruction leaflet of whichever preparation you are using.

Having done so, then get him to give an injection himself of a small dose (2.5 µg alprostadil or equivalent) with your guidance and assistance as necessary. Most men will have no problem with this. Some will find it totally impossible to mix the preparations and/or to inject it safely. If this is the case, it should probably be agreed that the treatment is not going to be suitable.

Beware the man who is tense and prone to syncope. Ask about any history of fainting attacks or needle phobia. You will need to be very careful in such a circumstance, as a vasovagal attack may be precipitated. It is best to demonstrate injections in such men when they are lying down. It is also sensible to have *atropine* available in the medicine cupboard. Such an event is very unusual but can occur.

Having determined that the man is safe, competent and prepared to try self-injection at home, doses should then be discussed. The potential problem of prolonged erections should be emphasised and discussed and written instructions given to him to keep in case such an event occurs (Table 6.3; Appendix III – this is only an example. *Any instructions must be discussed and agreed with the local urology department.*) It is extremely rare, provided that men use only the lowest effective dose required to produce an erection. The man should then be given written instructions for a gradually increasing incremental dose regime (Table 6.4).

Table 6.3 Suggested treatment procedure for prolonged erection

(1) A 25 gauge butterfly is inserted into one of the corpora;
(2) aspirate 50 ml of blood and apply pressure for 5 minutes;
(3) aspirate a further 50 ml if (2) fails, irrigate with heparinized saline and again apply pressure;
(4) if (3) fails, inject 200 µg of phenylephrine – repeat if (4) fails;
(5) if all measures fail, surgical treatment will be required.

Table 6.4 Instructions on dose of injection treatment

It is important that you use the lowest effective dose for you. It is difficult to predict what dose you will require, so I suggest that initially you start with a low dose and gradually increase until you find an effective one. This may take several separate attempts without success. You must never give a second dose within 24 hours even if the first did not work. This plan is essential to prevent you getting a prolonged erection which can be a serious problem (see below).

START WITH :

If no good next time try:

If no good next time try:

If no good next time try:

If no good next time try:

Doses will vary according to the agent used (see Table 6.5) but, if using alprostadil, a starting dose of 2.5 or 5 µg is reasonable. If ineffective, it should be increased to 10 µg, then 15 µg, then 20 µg. 40 µg preparations are also now available.

If patients require more than 40 µg, or if dosage is limited by painful side effects, there are a number of available options:

1. Use mixtures. Papaverine can be used instead of the normal diluent. This becomes an unlicensed mixture and informed consent/disclaimer may be sensible (see also Table 6.4).
2. Use ready made double or triple mixtures – either prepared by the pharmacy or as commercially available (e.g. vasoactive intestinal polypeptide (VIP)/phentolamine).

129

Table 6.5 Recommended doses of drugs for intracavernosal injection

Alprostadil: Starting dose 5–10 µg;
incremental increases by   5 µg up to 20 µg;
   10 µg up to 40 µg;
consider combination drugs if requirement > 40 µg.
Papaverine: Starting dose   10 mg;
incremental increases   5 mg up to 20 mg;
   10 mg up to 60 mg.

Combinations should start with combinations of minimum doses and increase by similar increments to those above. Combinations may also include phentolamine or VIP.

Other methods of initiating treatment

Other methods include the clinician giving the injections until a suitable dose is found in the clinic and then instructing the man on home self-injection. In my opinion this not only wastes time but may lead to prolonged erections. This is because the dose required to be effective in a sexually stimulating environment at home may be considerably lower than in the clinic.

The importance of instructing a man on the technique of intracavernosal injection should not necessarily to be to see if it is effective, but to see whether the man, and his supervising clinician, are happy that it will be safe and that the man will cope. Success will always only be determined by home use.

It may be useful to give men an instruction video to take home for reinforcement of the instructions given in the clinic.

If people are unsure, they should be allowed to borrow instruction videos of the various treatments to take home and discuss with their partner prior to deciding.

Follow-up arrangements

It is important to arrange some follow-up of patients to ensure that treatments are being managed satisfactorily, no local complications have occurred, and also for the purpose of audit and evaluation. Follow-up may be arranged in the diabetes clinic or within the separate erectile dysfunction clinic. Some follow-up can be done successfully by telephone, but it is essential to obtain consent and ensure the correct number and time of phoning is agreed. Otherwise, much embarrassment or worse could ensue.

Pharmaceuticals and prescribing

It will be necessary for an agreement to be reached with the pharmacy for the supply of all drugs that you are likely to use. It may be necessary to have this agreed by the local Drugs and Thera-peutics Committee. It is also important that there is agreement from primary care to provide further prescriptions and this may require agreement by the District Pharmaceutical Committee (or equivalent) for inclusion in formularies.

The amount of stock required will depend upon your prescribing policy and the numbers of patients seen. Even if the hospital policy is not to prescribe to outpatients, but to advise GPs, a small stock will still be required for demonstration and instruction purposes. It is most convenient if such a stock is kept in the diabetes unit itself. If the hospital does not provide prescriptions, it is useful to give patients a pretyped letter, concerning prescribing of the chosen treatment, to take to their GP to avoid delays in obtaining supplies.

Links with other disciplines

The majority of treatments can be managed by the diabetes care team, but there may be occasions when the assistance of urologists/androl-ogists or psychosexual specialists are required. It is useful therefore to establish links with a named department in these specialties. It is particularly important to obtain agreement with a local urology department regarding the advice given to patients on the action required should a prolonged erection occur.

There may be a local Relate Centre (previously Marriage Guidance Council) – see Appendix I – that it will be worth contacting regarding psychosexual aspects of the problem. It may be worth having their leaflets available in the clinic.

Educational requirements

Before establishing an erectile dysfunction service some initial and ongoing professional education will be required. It is worth visiting one or two established erectile failure clinics to obtain some experience in the process of running a clinic and particularly in observing the technique of intracavernosal injection treatment. For information on established clinics in the UK contact the Impotence Association (Appendix I).

Summary

Establishing an erectile dysfunction clinic is easy and rewarding. There are a variety of models that can be adopted. Few facilities are required and much of the work can be done by nurses or other health care professionals.

chapter 7

The role of the general practitioner

Patrick J Wright

Introduction

Until recently the management of erectile dysfunction has been the preserve of urologists, psychosexual counsellors and other hospital practitioners. It was not practical for most general practitioners (GPs) to provide treatments such as papaverine self-injection therapy or psychosexual counselling. As a result most patients were referred to secondary care. In recent years, however, new treatments including oral and transurethral therapy have become available; these are simpler to use and many GPs are now managing impotence in primary care. The publicity surrounding the advent of new treatments for erectile dysfunction has led to many more impotent men coming forward to seek help, and it is unlikely that secondary care alone can deal with the greatly increased demand.

There are challenges and advantages in the treatment of erectile dysfunction in general practice. A GP is more likely to know and understand a patient's particular circumstances. Impotent men may be less intimidated seeking help from their family practitioner than a hospital specialist or sexual therapist. Little specialised equipment is required, so there is no reason why interested GPs should not effectively treat the majority of men presenting with impotence.

A recent study aiming to investigate the role of the GP in the management of problems of sexual function revealed that the majority of GPs categorized sexual dysfunction as medium priority, with most doctors identifying common barriers to the management of sexual dysfunction. In practice, GPs' suggestions focused on the need for more professional and patient education, consultation time, psychosexual counsellors and relevant secondary care services.[1]

The prevalence of erectile dysfunction in general practice

The few studies of erectile dysfunction in general practice suggest it is an extremely common problem for which most men do not seek help. In a questionnaire survey of 170 patients attending a general practice, 31% of men experienced some form of sexual dysfunction and 17% experienced erectile dysfunction.[2] The vast majority of men (70%) considered it an appropriate problem to discuss with their GP but in only 2% of cases was it recorded in the patient's case notes. Of the 789 men who responded to a recent postal survey of 4000 adults registered with four general practices, 34% experienced sexual problems and 21.5% experienced erectile dysfunction.[3] Of the responders with a sexual problem, 52% said they would like professional help but only 10% had ever received such help.

A postal survey plus data extracted from patient records from 10 UK practices revealed a prevalence rate for ED of 52% with 39% reporting total ED. The results of a recent computer generated audit from my own UK 5 GP practice population are given in Table 7.1. Of the 160 male diabetic patients 37 have been assessed and have received treatment for their established ED.

Table 7.1

Males in pactice	4265
Males aged 25–79	2954
Males with ED	177
Males with ED and hypertension	43
Males with ED and diabetes	37
Males with ED and IHD	35
Males with ED and hypercholesterolaemia	15
Males with ED and depression	21
Males with ED and TURP	5
Maleswith ED and MS	2
Males with ED, diabetes and IHD	11
Males with ED, diabetes and hypertension	12
Males with ED, IHD and hypertension	7
Males with ED, diabetes, IHD and hypertension	5

ED, erectile dysfunction; TURP, transurethral resections of prostate; MS, multiple sclerosis; IHD, ischemic heart disease

Which patients in general practice are at risk of erectile dysfunction?

The prevalence of erectile dysfunction increases with age and is more common in men with coexisting medical problems, and it should be borne in mind that ED is associated with many types of drugs. The following conditions are associated with impotence, usually of organic association:[3,4]

- Hypertension and hypercholesterolaemia.
- Premature and generalised arteriopathy: especially if history of myocardial infarction or angina. (Also associated with advanced age and chronic smoking.)

- Diabetes mellitus.
- Iatrogenic factors, e.g. antihypertensive and antidepressant medication.
- Major abdominal, pelvic and prostate surgery.
- Miscellaneous causes: excess alcohol and obesity.
- Multiple sclerosis and spinal cord injury.
- Androgen deficiency. Surprisingly rare < 2%, yet still perceived by many men as a likely cause.[2,5]

The prevalence of predominantly psychogenic ED in primary care is less than for organic mediated ED, but should be suspected in the case of:

- sudden onset
- early collapse of erection
- good quality spontaneous erections when masturbating or waking
- premature ejaculation or inability to ejaculate
- relationship changes or problems
- major life events
- psychological problems
- coexistent depression or performance-related anxiety

It is unusual for any patient to have a single identifiable recognisable underlying causal factor – e.g. neurogenic, vasculogenic or psychogenic – even with specialist investigation.[6] Many men with organic related ED develop super-added performance-related anxiety which exacerbates their condition, resulting in mixed ED. A combination of medical and psychological treatment approaches may be necessary. It is more relevant for the attending practitioner to adopt a sympathetic and nonjudgmental approach to the patient and his partner and to respect their preferences for treatment than to try and determine the exactly aetiology of the erectile dysfunction.[7]

The management of erectile dysfunction in general practice

It is important to determine several key issues in order to make a more confident diagnosis:

1. How severe is his erectile dysfunction and how long has he had it?
2. What is the attitude of his partner or wife to this problem?
3. Are there any aggravating factors to consider such as stress or concomitant medication?

Assessment of erectile dysfunction in primary care

In keeping with the numerous and wide ranging conditions that GPs encounter on a day-to-day basis, the GP may choose to gather the relevant information from the history and perform the appropriate examination and investigations during a series of consultations with the patient. Some GPs may find it helpful to issue the patient with a leaflet or questionnaire as an aid for information gathering during initial assessment, thus saving time for discussion about partnership issues and treatment options, and for gauging progress at subsequent consultations. Patient information and advice leaflets can be downloaded from the Impotence Association at www.impotence.org.uk.

Other GPs may choose to refer their patients to a fellow partner or colleague with a particular interest in erectile dysfunction or to their practice nurse, who may have received appropriate training in the assessment of patients with erectile dysfunction. This decision may be influenced by the severity of the ED together with the presence of co-morbidities, e.g. cardiac disease or diabetes mellitus.

If possible, the partner's medical history should also be explored as she may also be suffering from sexual problem. A recent study of couples consulting about ED revealed that at least half the couples had not experienced any sexual activity in 2.5 years and whereas 87% of men considered intercourse important, only 20% of the women rated intercourse somewhat or very important.

If time permits, asking some of the following six key questions may facilitate adopting a more structured approach to the assessment.

Six key questions: a general practitioner aid for assessing the severity of erectile dysfunction[8]

1   What is the problem with your erections?

Useful cues:
- How did it start?
- Consider both initial degree of firmness and ability to maintain firmness allowing penetrative sexual intercourse (as a percentage of attempts at intercourse that were satisfactory).
- Degree of firmness.
- Presence or absence of early morning, nocturnal or spontaneous erections.
- Ability to still achieve orgasm and ejaculation.

2   How long has there been a problem?

Useful cues:
- Abrupt suggests psychogenic causation.
- Gradual onset suggests organic causation.

3   Do you regard your sex drive (libido) as being normal?

Useful cues:
- Compared with say 5 years ago?
- Lowered libido could reflect significantly reduced androgen levels, although anxiety and depression are more probable causes, e.g. patients with established ED may anticipate 'failure' and therefore seek to avoid sexual relations with their partners.

4 What is the attitude of your partner towards your problem?

Useful cues:

- Try and gain insight into the quality of the relationship.
- Try to establish if there is any underlying performance anxiety.
- and is this a primary or secondary effect of the erectile ED?

5 What do you think is causing your erections to fail and have you and your partner done anything about it?

Useful cues:

- Worth sharing views on possible iatrogenic factors with a temporal association with onset of erectile difficulties.
- Worth knowing if the patient has already sought advice or obtained any treatment before consulting with you.

6 What are you and your partner hoping to gain from any treatments that might be available?

Useful cues:

- A chance to assess your patient's expectations from treatments on offer.
- Consider whether these are realistic or unattainable.

Examination

For the majority of patients, examination should be limited to the basic minimum—that is blood pressure and examination of the genitalia (to include checking for abnormalities of testicular size, fibrosis of penile shaft, and retractable foreskin.) Further examination may be appropriate where indicated by age or findings in the history-especially regarding cardiovascular, neurological, endocrine and urinary systems.

The important aspects of the physical examination include:[8]

- blood pressure
- genitalia (testicular volume, exclude Peyronie's disease and phimosis)
- lower limb reflexes*
- peripheral pulses*
- gynaecomastia*
- digital rectal examination*.

*Only if clinically indicated.

Investigations

Essential investigations should include a fasting venous plasma glucose estimation to exclude Diabetes Mellitus or impaired glucose tolerance. Precise investigations will depend on the history and examination findings:

- Fasting serum cholesterol if vasculogenic cause suspected.
- Early morning serum serum testosterone and prolactin levels if the history or examination suggests possible hypogonadism, loss of libido in younger patients or if required to reassure patients.
- Luteinising hormone level if testosterone low.
- Thyroid function studies if suspected thyoid disorder.
- Liver function studies if suspected liver disorder.
- Renal function studies if suspected renal impairment.
- Prostate Specific Antigen assay in men over 50 with predominant lower urinary tract symptoms or as a base line in patients who are to receive androgen replacement therapy.
- To exclude lower urinary tract disorder.

Treatment options for erectile dysfunction in general practice

Lifestyle factors

When a man presents with erectile dysfunction, his GP has an opportunity to consider other health issues and screen for underlying causes.

140

Erectile dysfunction is often associated with asymptomatic conditions that benefit from early detection, such as diabetes, hypertension and hyperlipidaemia. It is therefore important to consider general health issues and to address lifestyle factors. Therefore, advice should be given on smoking, alcohol intake, obesity and lack of exercise as appropriate. However, these should not be used as an excuse for not offering an effective treatment for erectile dysfunction. For patients with coexistent or previously documented cardiac disease or cerebrovascular accident, an appraisal of the patient's current exercise tolerance and concomitant medication is essential as the majority of patients with cardiac disease will be at low or intermediate cardiac risk and can be safely and effectively managed in primary care.[10] Heart disease itself is not a contraindication; however, sexual dysfunction is an important problem in the context of cardiovascular disease. All current available treatments for impotence are suitable for a cardiovascular patient and if used according to the instructions, do not increase the cardiac risk.[10]

Patients considered at greater risk, e.g. poor effort tolerance and dependent on regular use of nitrates might require a cardiological assessment prior to initiating treatment in primary care.

Psychosexual counselling (via suitably accredited counsellor)

Main indications
A dysfunctional relationship or severe psychogenic impotence.[11]

Advantages
- No drug treatment usually required.
- Partner usually involved in the treatment programme.
- Change in behaviour and attitudes can lead to a lasting cure (but rarely in diabetic men).

Disadvantages
- Locally based service often patchy and inadequately resourced.
- Often relies on patient self-funding and many cannot afford this.

- Patients are often reluctant to attend either alone or with their partners.
- Time-consuming.
- Rarely effective when used alone in diabetic men.

Oral therapy

Sildenafil and apomorphine

Sildenafil (Viagra) and Apomorphine SL (Uprima) are the two licensed, oral treatments for ED currently available in Europe and are the first line therapies for most men. The modes of action of these two drugs differ – apomorphine acts centrally to initiate the erection process by stimulating dopamine receptors in the paraventricular nucleus in the brain, while sildenafil acts peripherally on the penile vasculature and for this reason it is worth trying the alternative drug if one has failed in an individual patient.

Both drugs require adequate stimulation to produce an erection. Onset of action may be faster with apomorphine's sublingual formulation: it begins working, on average, within 20 minutes of administration compared with 30–60 minutes with sildenafil tablets, whose absorption may be affected by intake of large or fatty meals. Although the results of comparative studies for these drugs currently in progress are awaited, overall a more efficacious response to sildenafil seems likely, based on a higher percentage of reported intercourse rates among similar groups of patients who kept diary recordings during numerous clinical trials.

The beneficial effect was seen in many sub-groups of patients including those patients with organic illnesses, such as:

- Hypertension
- Ischaemic heart disorder
- Diabetes
- Neurological disease
- Abdominal and pelvic surgery
- Depression
- Psychogenic causality.

Due to age related changes in pharmacokinetics, dosage adjustment is required for older men taking sildenafil from an initial dosage of 25 mg titrated to 50 mg or 100 mg. Younger men < 65 years may be initiated at a dosage of 50 mg. Apomorphine is normally initiated at a dose of 2 mg then titrated up to 3 mg in the majority of patients.

For patients with established ischaemic heart disease taking oral nitrates apomorphine can be coprescribed with caution. Nitrates are an absolute contraindication for the use of sildenafil. Yet patients with adequate effort tolerance and with little or no need for use of glyceryl trinitrate spray (GTN Spray) during exertion (i.e. mild stable angina) may take sildenafil but should be instructed not to use a GTN spray within 24 hours of taking sildenafil. For those patients considered too unfit to resume sexual activity a cardiologists opinion should be sought.

For adverse effects with apomorphine SL reported in clinical trials, see Table 7.1.

Table 7.1

	Apomorphine 3 mg (%)	Placebo %
Nausea	7	1.1
Yawning	8.1	0.6
Dizziness	6.5	3.4
Somnolence	4.9	1.7
Headache	2.2	4.5
Vasodilation	2.2	2.3

Headache was also experienced by clinical trial patients taking sildenafil 13%, while other adverse effects include flushing 10% altered vision 2% and dyspepsia 7%.

Advantages
- Oral medications widely accepted by the majority of erectile dysfunction patients.

- Many GPs feel more comfortable prescribing oral agents.
- Efficacy rates reported between 50 and 90%.
- Noninvasive.
- Side effects transient and mild.

Disadvantages
- Facilitator rather than initiator of erections.
- Slower onset of action than injected alprostadil.

Sildenafil is also contraindicated in patients with severe hepatic impairment, hypotension, hereditary degenerative retinal disorders, and recent stroke or myocardial infarction.

Transurethral alprostadil[12]

Advantages
- Simple delivery method – no needles.
- Variable reported efficacy rates between 30 and 70%.
- Extremely low risk of priapism and fibrosis.

Disadvantages
- Long-term safety uncertain.
- High incidence of local discomfort and burning sensation.
- Technically too demanding and unacceptable for some.
- Variable efficacy.
- More expensive than oral and injection therapies.

Absolute contraindications
As for injection therapy; also urethritis/balanitis.
Use of condom recommended if partner is pregnant.

Intracorporeal injection therapy

Main indications
Moderate to severe erectile dysfunction due to any cause.[13]

Advantages
- Modern delivery systems with ultra-fine needles acceptable to the majority of severe sufferers and partners.
- Modern treatments associated with good efficacy rates and lower incidence of side effects including priapism.
- Available on prescription from GP.
- Rapid onset of action following injection mimics natural erection response.

Disadvantages
- Side effects unacceptable to some.
- Many GPs have no experience of using it and are reluctant to start.
- Regarded as costly by many. Some GPs are reluctant to prescribe it and rationing is not uncommon.
- High dropout rates reported, over 1 year > 50% in many studies.
- Can be technically demanding for some patients with morbid obesity, poor coordination or poor vision.

Absolute contraindications
Increased clotting tendency or penile fibrosis.

Any GP considering offering treatment for erectile dysfunction must warn his patients of the possibility of priapism and advise them of a plan of action if it occurs. Usually this would involve advising the patient to attend his local Accident and Emergency Department if an erection lasts more than 4 hours. It is often useful to advise them to take the leaflet provided by the manufacturers to show the doctor at the hospital.

Vacuum tumescence therapy

Main indications
Moderate to severe erectile dysfunction due to any cause.[14]

Advantages
- No drug treatment required.
- Very cost-effective if used over a long period of time.
- No risk of drug interactions.

Disadvantages
- Many couples find the method cumbersome, contrived and unacceptable.
- Initial capital outlay (price range £90–200) unacceptable for some patients.
- Erection is cooler and pivots at base.
- Tension ring causes some discomfort.

Absolute contraindications
Anticoagulation therapy.

Androgen therapy
Endocrine causes for erectile dysfunction are uncommon and require specialist assessment. It would be unwise to initiate androgen therapy for erectile dysfunction or loss of libido, and if a genuine case of androgen deficiency is suspected, referral to an endocrinologist is recommended.

Reviewing patients with erectile dysfunction in primary care
Encouraging flexible arrangement of follow-up for patients who have been assessed and treated in primary care is rewarding and in keeping with other complex conditions frequently managed in primary care such as irritable bowel syndrome, migraine and dyspepsia. The aims are to ensure the intervention is proving efficacious and safe and to address any issues the patient may have in relation to his erectile dysfunction. Efficacy of treatment will depend on:

- treating only those patients who truly have erectile dysfunction
- using the treatment most appropriate for the individual
- continuing treatment only if it is effective

■ supporting discontinuation of treatment if a consistent recovery of spontaneous erection occurs.

Urology referral

Some patients with erectile dysfunction may fail to respond to conventional treatments as outlined above. Some of these may be considered as suitable candidates for insertion of a penile prosthesis. However, not many are willing to consider surgery, as they may perceive that the potential risks outweigh the potential benefits.[10] Those patients who are willing to consider this method of treatment must undergo intensive counselling, as appropriate case selection is crucial in determining the long-term success rate. In the United Kingdom many health authorities now limit the number of such procedures carried out, since the implementation of the schedule 11 guidelines for erectile dysfunction treatment (see below). However, those patients with severe Peyronie's disease and erectile dysfunction may benefit from surgical intervention for correction of the penile deformity, which may be hampering the patient's ability to overcome their erectile dysfunction by conventional means.[10]

Although there are no randomised trials comparing the cost effectiveness of management in primary or secondary care, patients can be managed with confidence, at least initially in primary care. Indeed, recently published guidelines incorporating new treatments and current views have been synthesized by a multi-disciplinary panel of experts. They are written with the primary care team in mind and may also be helpful to doctors working in other disciplines.[14,15]

Using the team in general practice

There is a long tradition in general practice of using a multidisciplinary team approach to manage a variety of chronic diseases. General Practitioners are therefore well placed to take on the management of erectile dysfunction with the support of their colleagues from other disciplines. With appropriate educational support, many well-motivated practice nurses are capable of developing a counselling role for male patients who first raise the subject of erectile dysfunction with them.

They are particularly well placed in their diabetic, hypertension, cardiovascular and well man mini-clinics to identify patients with erectile dysfunction. Some patients may perceive them as being less pressurised than their GP colleagues. Many practice nurses find it helpful to use a preassessment template to assist with recording of essential information in chronological order from the patient's history. Several pharmaceutical companies are willing to offer free educational training support and materials for both GPs and practice nurses involved with patients with erectile dysfunction.

What audit or survey might be conducted in the practice?
Many formal trials of erectile dysfunction treatments were done using hospital patient populations, which are perhaps not representative of the type of patients seen in everyday practice. It is therefore important that GPs audit their results to determine the efficacy of the treatments being used. The topics to be audited might include:

■ Run computerised audit on the practice disease index to determine numbers of patients with impotence. (Match these cases with concomitant medical conditions and run a check on concomitant medication for possible associations with the erectile dysfunction.)
■ Audit referral patterns for this group of patients.
■ Audit prescribing data for this group: e.g. to determine preferred treatments.
■ Audit prescribing costs for the group overall.

Screening for erectile dysfunction in general practice
Drawing an analogy to the female menopause, it is of interest to consider how active members of the team should be in raising the subject of erectile dysfunction with our patients. Many impotent men would like treatment but are reluctant to ask. Do we wait until our patients (or their partners) raise the subject or should we be proactive and discuss the issue with those patients in at-risk groups? In

an ideal world with unlimited resources the answer would probably be yes. Unfortunately, resources are limited and screening for erectile dysfunction in at-risk groups would undoubtedly result in an increase in workload for GPs, with identification of greater numbers of patients and subsequent counselling with a view to providing treatment. Currently, when a GP or practice nurse is faced with a patient with a high risk of having erectile dysfunction, he will have to make a judgement on an individual basis in light of the time and resources available.

Rationing of therapies for erectile dysfunction

In an unprecedented move the UK government introduced changes in June 1999 to limit a potential rise in National Health Service (NHS) prescribing costs for erectile dysfunction treatments by restricting NHS treatments to certain categories of patients (see Chapter 4). This was achieved by making treatment for erectile dysfunction part of 'schedule 11'. Fortunately for diabetologists and GPs treating diabetic men, diabetes was included in the list of conditions for which erectile dysfunction treatment could be prescribed on the NHS. The full list of conditions is given in Table 4.7.

Conclusion

The launch of more effective and safe therapies and increased public awareness of erectile dysfunction has resulted in GPs seeing increased numbers of patients seeking treatment for the condition. Inevitably, there has been a shift from the traditional secondary care across to primary care for the management of these patients. Indeed, erectile dysfunction is a health problem well suited to management in a primary care setting. Most GPs already possess knowledge and skills required to deliver high standards of care accessible to affected men and couples. However, not all GPs are enthusiastic about assessing patients (and their partners). Many perceive it as a potentially costly and time-consuming process that which lacks the financial incentive of the 'item for service payments' which is applied to the more traditional tasks currently undertaken in primary care. Despite advances in treatments for erectile dysfunction, members of the primary care team and the public need better information and support in order to succeed in delivering effective treatment safely to those with the greatest needs.

References

1. Humphrey S, Nazareth I. GP's views on their management of sexual dysfunction. Fam Pract 2001; 18:516–8.
2. Read S, King M, Watson J. Sexual dysfunction in primary medical care: prevalence, characteristics and detection by the general practitioner. J Public Health Med 1997; 19(4):387–91.
3. Dunn KM, Croft PR, Hackett GI. Sexual problems: a study of the prevalence and need for health care in the general population. Fam Pract 1998; 15(6):519–24.
4. Korenman SG. Advances in the understanding and management of erectile dysfunction. J Clin Endocrinol Metab 1995; 60:1985–8.
5. Feldman HA, Goldstein I. Impotence and its medical and psychosocial correlates. Results of the Massachusetts Male Aging Study. J Urol 1994; 151:54–61.
6. Krane RJ. Impotence. N Engl J Med 1989; 321:1648–9.
7. Carrier S, Zvara P, Lue T. Erectile dysfunction. Endocrinol Metab Clin N Am 1994; 23:773–82.
8. O'Keefe M, Hunt DK. Assessment and treatment of impotence. Med Clin N Am 1995; 79:415–34.
9. Kirby RS. Impotence: diagnosis and management of male erectile dysfunction. Br Med J 1994; 308:957–61.
10. Wright P. Impotence: the GP's role. Update 8th April 1998, 615–24.
11. Wagner G. Update on male erectile dysfunction. Clinical Review. Br Med J 1998; 7132:678–82.
12. Padma-Nathan H. Treatment of men with erectile dysfunction with transurethral alprostadil. Medicated urethral system for erection (MUSE) study group. N Eng J Med 1997; 336:1–7.
13. Linet OI. Efficacy and safety of intracavernosal alprostadil in men with erectile dysfunction. N Engl J Med 1996; 334:873–7.
14. Ralph D, McNicholas T. UK management guidelines for erectile dysfunction. Br Med J 2000; 7259. 321:499–503.
15. Riley A, Wright P, Ralph D, Russell I. Guidelines for the management of erectile dysfunction. Trends Urol Gynaecol Sexual Health 2002; 7(2).

International Index of Erectile Function (IIEF) erectile domain questionnaire

How often were you able to get an erection during sexual activity?

0 = no sexual activity

1 = almost never/never

2 = a few times (much less than half the time)

3 = sometimes (about half the time)

4 = most of the time (much more than half the time)

5 = almost always/always

When you had erections with sexual stimulation, how often were your erections hard enough for penetration?

0 = no sexual activity

1 = almost never/never

2 = a few times (much less than half the time)

3 = sometimes (about half the time)

4 = most of the time (much more than half the time)

5 = almost always/always

When you attempted sexual intercourse how often were you able to penetrate (enter) your partner?

0 = did not attempt intercourse

1 = almost never/never

2 = a few times (much less than half the time)

3 = sometimes (about half the time)

4 = most times (much more than half the time)

5 = almost always/always

During sexual intercourse how often were you able to maintain your erection after you had penetrated (entered) your partner?

0 = did not attempt intercourse

1 = almost never/never

2 = a few times (much less than half the time)

3 = sometimes (about half the time)

4 = most times (much more than half the time)

5 = almost always/always

During sexual intercourse how difficult was it to maintain your erection to completion of intercourse

0 = did not attempt intercourse

1 = extremely difficult

2 = very difficult

3 = difficult

4 = slightly difficult

5 = not difficult

How do you rate your confidence that you could get and keep an erection?

1 = very low

2 = low

3 = moderate

4 = high

5 = very high

ERECTILE FAILURE PRO FORMA:

Name   Date
Address

Post Code   GP

PROBLEM:
1. ERECTIONS:
   Failure obtain / sustain   Onset: Sudden / Gradual
   Partial / Complete failure   Duration of problem:
   Nocturnal Yes / No   Spontaneous Yes / No
                                   Masturbation Yes / No
   Partner Yes / No   Single Yes / No
   Intercourse: Occasional / Never / Last time =

2. EJACULATION:
   Normal / Retro / Quick / None.   ORGASM: Yes / No

3. LIBIDO: Normal / Reduced.

4. RELATIONSHIP: PSYCHOLOGY:

OTHER CONDiTIONS:

Diabetes: NIDDM / IDDM.   Duration =   Rx:

Microvascular disease: Yes / No

Vascular: IHD: Yes / No   PVD: Yes / No

CVD: Yes / No   Cigs: Yes / No

Dyslipidaemia: Yes / No   Hypertension: Yes / No   Rx:

Neurological:

Psychiatric / Psychological: Comments:

Urological:

Peyronies: Yes / No

MEDICATIONS:

CAUSE:

Congenital:

Acquired: Organic / Psychological / Mixed O+P / Mixed P+O

Organic =

EXAMINATION: Penis: Testes: Prostate:

INVESTIGATIONS: Testosterone: Total: Androgen Index:

                                     Free: DHEAs

                     Prolactin

                     PSA

                     Other:

TREATMENT: Initial   Subsequent (date)

                                      1   2   3   4

Oral:

Vacuum Device: Type:

Self-injection: Type:

MUSE:

Psychosexual:

None:

Other:

Seen By: **Date:**   **Review:**

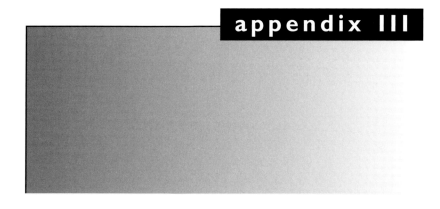

INSTRUCTIONS IF PROLONGED ERECTION OCCURS

In the rare event of an erection lasting more than 4 hours and assuming you have tried "sexual activity", make every attempt you can think of to get rid of it!

This might include:

1. Try vigorous leg exercise. Either on an exercise bicycle / machine or running / cycling.

2. Try ice packs, frozen peas or whatever is to hand.

3. If ineffective try again after a further 1 and 2 hours.

4. If despite these attempts to get rid of it the erection still persists 6 hours after the injection YOU MUST GO TO YOUR LOCAL CASUALTY DEPARTMENT WITHOUT FURTHER DELAY, EVEN IF IT IS THE MIDDLE OF THE NIGHT. IT IS EASY FOR THEM TO CORRECT THE PROBLEM IF YOU GO EARLY ENOUGH. IF YOU DELAY BEYOND 8 HOURS YOU MAY REQUIRE A DIFFICULT OPERATION.

   TAKE THIS FORM AND ACCOMPANYING INSTRUCTIONS FOR DOCTORS WITH YOU.

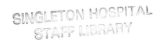

6. Contact me before giving further injections so that we can discuss dosage and technique.

DEAR DOCTOR:

This patient has been instructed by me on the technique of intra-cavernosal self-injection therapy for erectile failure. He has now developed a prolonged erection unresponsive to the above measures.

I would be grateful if you would consider this as a matter of urgency and follow the enclosed instructions, or your own protocol, to help him get rid of the prolonged erection.

Thank you for your attention and I apologise for any inconvenience.

Dr William Alexander FRCP
Consultant Physician. Diabetes Unit.

PROTOCOL FOR TREATMENT OF
PHARMACOLOGICALLY INDUCED PRIAPISM

Many men with erectile failure are now successfully using intracorporeal self-injection therapy with vasoactive drugs. Rarely this treatment may cause prolonged erections and men are asked to attend for detumescence if erection persist beyond 6 hours.

IT IS ESSENTIAL THAT THIS PROBLEM IS TREATED URGENTLY.

SUGGESTED TREATMENT PROTOCOL:

ASPIRATION

Using aseptic technique, insert a 19–21 gauge butterly needle (or equivalent) into the corpus cavernosum and aspirate 25–50 mIs of blood. If detumescence not produced then repeat the procedure on the other side.

If unsuccessful then local alpha-adrenergic medication is recommended.

ALPHA-ADRENERIC INTRACORPOREAL INJECTION

- Make up a 200 microgram/mI solution of phenylephrine in a 5 ml syringe (1 mg total).
- Inject 0.5–I mI of the solution into one corpora every 5–10 minutes and massage to spread the drug.
- The maximum dose of phenylephrine is 1 mg – (5 mIs of the 200 microgram/mI solution).
- If necessary further aspiration of 25–50 mls of blood can then also be tried through the same butterfly needle.
- MONITOR BP AND PULSE THROUGHOUT AS POTENTIAl HYPERTENSIVE CRISIS CAN OCCUR.
- CAUTION – IF PATIENT IS ON MONOAMINE OXIDASE INHIBITORS
  - IF PATIENT HYPERTENSIVE
  - IF CORONARY OR CEREBRAL ARTERY DISEASE

IF ABOVE FAILS
URGENT SURGICAL REFERRAL TO UROLOGY FOR FURTHER MANAGEMENT WHICH MAY ENTAIL A SHUNT PROCEDURE.

Useful organisations

British Association of Sexual and Relationship Therapy

http://www.basmt.org.uk/

British Society for Sexual and Impotence Research (BSSIR)

http://www.bssir.com/

Greystones

113 Whitchurch Road

Tavistock

Devon PL19 9BQ

Tel: 01822 610260

Diabetes UK (formerly the British Diabetic Association)

http://www.diabetes.org.uk/home.htm

Diabetes UK Central Office

10 Parkway

London NW1 7AA

Tel: 020 7323 1531

Fax: 020 7637 3644

European Society of Impotence Research (ESIR)

http://www.essir.net/

Antonio Robles no 4 (9C)

Madrid 28034

Spain

Tel: +34 91 358 3854

Fax: +34 91 358 5045

Impotence Association
http://www.impotence.org.uk/
P.O. Box 10296
London SW17 9WH
Tel: 020 8767 7791 (Helpline)

International Society of Impotence Research (ISIR)
http://www.urolog.nl/artsen/isir/index.htm
P.O. Box 97
3950 AB MAARN
The Netherlands
Tel. +31 343 443888
Fax. +31 343 442043

Relate (Formerly the Marriage Guidance Council)
http://www.relate.org.uk/
Herbert Gray College
Little Church Street
Rugby
Warwickshire CV21 3AP
Tel: 01788 573241

Index

Note: references to figures are indicated by 'f' and references to tables by 't' when they fall on a page not covered by the text reference

acetylcholine, in erection 18, 21–2
adrenergic mechanisms of erection
   18–20
   see also cholinergic mechanisms
afferent nerves 14
age factor 56–7
alprostadil (prostaglandin E_1)
   intracavernosal 85–9, 130
   transurethral 90, 91f, 144
   see also prostaglandins
American Urological Association
   Inc., Erectile Dysfunction
   Clinical Guidelines Panel 115–16
androgens 31–2
   oral therapy 91, 146
angiopathy, diabetic 36–7
antihypertensive agents 40, 75t, 76
apomorphine 92–3, 142–3
arterial revascularization 118
arteriogenic impotence 37
audit in general practice 147–8
autonomic nervous system,
   dysfunction 70–1
awareness programmes 61, 122

Brindley, G S 84
British Association of Sexual and
   Relationship Therapy 159
British Diabetic Association (BDA)
   see Diabetes UK
British Society for Sexual and
   Impotence Research (BSSIR) 159

calcitonin gene-related peptide 27–8
calcium 30–1
cardiovascular disease 38–9, 97–8, 141
cholinergic mechanisms of erection
   21–2
   see also adrenergic mechanisms
clinics, organisation 121–32
   consultation 125–30
   follow-up 131
   structure 122–5
Cooper Clinic (Dallas) Study 42
corpus cavernosum 10–12, 13, 16
   adrenergic mechanisms 19–20
   cholinergic mechanisms 21
   see also intracavernosal injection
      therapy

corpus spongiosum 10, 11f, 14, 16
  adrenergic mechanisms 19
  cholinergic mechanisms 21
counselling 74–8
  psychosexual 77–8, 141–2
cyclic adenosine monophosphate
  (cAMP) 25, 30
cyclic guanosine monophosphate
  (cGMP) 24, 30, 33, 95f

diabetes care services and erectile
  dysfunction 59, 60, 65–6,
  121–32
Diabetes UK (formerly British
  Diabetic Association) 5, 60, 159
diabetic angiopathy 36–7
diabetic neuropathy 36–7, 70–1
drugs
  cause of erectile dysfunction 40,
  75t, 76
  prescribing 131
  rationing 99, 100t, 148

efferent nerves 14–16
endocrine function, investigation
  71–3
endothelins, in erection 29–30
endothelium, in erection 23–5, 36–7,
  38–9
Erecaid 78–9, 80
erectile dysfunction
  aetiology 4–5, 33–42, 64–5, 72t
    in general practice 134–6
    medication and drugs 75t, 76
  assessment 61–5, 69–74, 123–4,
  125–31
    in general practice 137–9
  attitudes 3–6
  cardiovascular disease 38–9
  clinical history 62–5
  clinics, organisation 121–32

counselling 74–8, 77–8, 141–2
  defined 2
  epidemiology 55–61, 134–6
  investigations 69–74, 140
  management 69–101, 126–30
    general practice 133–49
  neurogenic 41
  neuropathy, diabetic 36–7, 70–1
  pathophysiology 33–42
  physical examination 65, 139–40
  physical treatments 78–84, 126–30
  risk factors 135–6
  surgical treatment 109–18, 146–7
  vasculogenic 37
Erectile Dysfunction Clinical
  Guidelines Panel, American
  Urological Association
  Inc.115–16
erection
  haemodynamics 16–18
  neurophysiology 18–33
  nocturnal 69–70
  pharmacology 18–33
  physiology 9–10, 16–33
  prolonged 87–8, 128, 145, 155–7
  spontaneous 69–70
  spontaneous return 96
European Society of Impotence
  Research (ESIR) 159

follow-up of patients 131, 146

general practice, management of
  erectile dysfunction 133–49
  assessment 137–9
  audit 147–8
  epidemiology 134–6
  examination 139–40
  investigation 140
  screening 148
  treatment 140–7

gonadal function, investigation 71–3
guanosine triphosphate (GTP) 95f

histamine 28–9
hypertension, risk factor for erectile
    dysfunction 39, 135
hypogonadism 71–3

impotence *see* erectile dysfunction
Impotence Association 56, 59, 137, 160
International Index of Erectile
    Function (IIEF) questionnaire
    124, 151–2
International Society of Impotence
    Research (ISIR) 160
intracavernosal injection
    investigation 71
    therapy 83–9, 90, 127–30, 144–5
    see also corpus cavernosum
Invicorp 89

ketanserin 20
Kinsey report 56

libido 31, 62–3, 72, 138
lifestyle factors 140–1

Marriage Guidance Council *see*
    Relate
Massachusetts Male Aging Study 42,
    56
Masters WH & Johnson V E 4,
    76–7
masturbation 3–4
Medicated Urethral System for
    Erection (MUSE) 90, 91f
medication, cause of erectile
    dysfunction 40, 75t, 76
muscarinic receptors 21, 22
MUSE (Medicated Urethral System
    for Erection) 90, 91f

Nesbit procedure 116–17
neurogenic erectile dysfunction 41
neuronal function, investigation 70–1
neuropathy, diabetic 36–7, 70–1
neuropeptide Y 27
neurotransmitters in erection 18–33
    adrenergic mechanisms 18–20
    cholinergic mechanisms 21–2
    nitric oxide 23–5
    second messengers 30–1, 32f
    sex hormones 31–2
nitrate therapy and sildenafil 98
nitric oxide 18, 23–5, 38, 95f
non-adrenergic non-cholinergic
    (NANC) transmission 22, 95f
noradrenaline 18–20, 22

occlusive vascular disease 37
oral therapy 91–101, 126, 142–3
    rationing 99, 100t, 148

papaverine 84–9, 129–30
parasympathetic nervous system
    14–16, 21–2
    see also sympathetic nervous
        system
patient aids 125
patient information 137
penile erection *see* erection
penile prosthesis implantation
    109–16, 146–7
penis
    anatomy 10–16
    erection *see* erection
    fibrosis 88
    pain 88, 90
Peyronie's disease 116–17, 147
phentolamine 84–5, 89, 92
phenylephrine 19
phosphodiesterase (PDE) 5
    inhibitors 93–101

potassium 31
priapism 87–8, 128, 145, 155–7
primary care, management of
    erectile dysfunction *see* general
    practice, management of
    erectile dysfunction
prostaglandins 25–7
  and smoking 41–2
  see also alprostadil
psychosexual counselling 77–8,
    141–2

quality of life 59–60, 87
questionnaires, assessment 124

Relate (formerly Marriage Guidance
    Council) 132, 160
relationships, effect of erectile
    dysfunction on 59–60, 74,
    138–9
renal failure 40–1
RigiScan 70

Saenz deTejada, I S 38
screening 60–1, 122–3, 149
second messengers in erection 30–1,
    32f
self-injection therapy 83–9, 90,
    127–30, 144–5
sex hormones in erection 31–2
sexual function, attitudes to 2–3
sexual relations 137–8, 138–9
sildenafil (Viagra) 94–9, 101f, 142–3
smoking 41–2, 76
smooth muscle in erection 16–18
  corporeal 11–12, 19–20, 24, 30–1,
    32f

Stekel, Wilhelm 4
substance P 28
surgical treatment 109–18, 146–7
sympathetic nervous system 14–16,
    18–20
    see also parasympathetic nervous
        system

tadalafil 99–100, 101f
testosterone 31–2, 91
topical treatment 93, 126
transurethral alprostadil 90, 91f, 127,
    144
trazodone 20, 93

uprima 142
urology referral 146–7

vacuum therapy 78–84, 126, 145–6
vardenafil 100, 101f
vascular function, assessment 70
vasculogenic erectile dysfunction 37
vasoactive intestinal polypeptide
    (VIP) 22, 25, 89
vasoconstriction 32f
Vasomax 92
vasorelaxation 32f
veno-corporeal incompetence 39–40,
    117–18
veno-occlusion in erection 17–18,
    37, 39–40, 70
venous leak *see* veno-corporeal
    incompetence
Viagra 94–9, 101f, 142–3
Virag, R 84

yohimbine 91–2